Modern Methods
in Medical Microbiology
Systems and Trends

Proceedings of the Sixth Annual Symposium of the Eastern Pennsylvania Branch of the American Society for Microbiology, Philadelphia, 14–15 November 1974

PROGRAM CHAIRMAN: Vern Pidcoe, Dr. P.H.

SYMPOSIUM CHAIRMAN: Jay E. Satz, Ph.D.

SYMPOSIUM SPONSORS:

Eastern Pennsylvania Branch, American Society for Microbiology, Philadelphia, Pennsylvania

Bureau of Laboratories, Pennsylvania Department of Health, Philadelphia, Pennsylvania

Department of Microbiology, Hahnemann Medical College and Hospital, Philadelphia, Pennsylvania

Department of Microbiology and Immunology, Temple University Health Sciences Center, Philadelphia, Pennsylvania

CONTRIBUTORS:

CIBA-GEIGY Corp.
Summit, New Jersey

Cooke Laboratory Products
A division of Dynatech Laboratory, Inc.
Alexandria, Virginia

Flow Laboratories, Inc.
Rockville, Maryland

Forma Scientific, Inc.
Marietta, Ohio

Merck, Sharpe, and Dohme
West Point, Pennsylvania

Schering Corp.
Bloomfield, New Jersey

Previously published volumes in the series of symposia sponsored by the Eastern Pennsylvania Branch of the American Society for Microbiology:

AUSTRALIA ANTIGEN (Proceedings of the Third Annual Symposium, edited by James E. Prier and Herman Friedman)

OPPORTUNISTIC PATHOGENS (Proceedings of the Fourth Annual Symposium, edited by James E. Prier and Herman Friedman)

QUALITY CONTROL IN MICROBIOLOGY (Proceedings of the Fifth Annual Symposium, edited by James E. Prier, Josephine T. Bartola, and Herman Friedman)

Modern Methods in Medical Microbiology
Systems and Trends

Edited by

James E. Prier, D.V.M., Ph.D
Josephine T. Bartola, M.Ed., J.D.
Herman Friedman, Ph.D

University Park Press
Baltimore · London · Tokyo

UNIVERSITY PARK PRESS
International Publishers in Science and Medicine
Chamber of Commerce Building
Baltimore, Maryland 21202

Typeset by The Composing Room of Michigan, Inc.

Manufactured in the United States of America by Universal Lithographers,
Inc., and the Maple Press Co.

Library of Congress Cataloging in Publication Data
Main entry under title:

Modern methods in medical microbiology.

   Proceedings of the symposium, Modern methods in
medical microbiology: systems and trends, sponsored
by the Eastern Pennsylvania Branch of the American
Society for Microbiology, and others, which was held
in Philadelphia, Nov. 14-15, 1974.
   1. Medical microbiology—Technique—Congresses.
I. Prier, James E. II. Bartola, Josephine T.
III. Friedman, Herman, 1931-   IV. American Society
for Microbiology. Eastern Pennsylvania Branch.
[DNLM: 1. Bacteriological technics—Congresses.
2. Microbiology—Methods—Congresses. QW25 S989m 1974]

QR46.M66   616.01'028   75-35795
ISBN 0-8391-0862-1

Contents

Participants   ix

Symposium Keynote Address: Recent and Future Changes in the
Clinical Microbiology Laboratory *John C. Sherris*   xiii

Section I   The Increased Role of Regulatory Agencies in Microbiology

    Introduction *James E. Prier*   3

       Chapter 1   Food and Drug Administration Regulation of in
Vitro Diagnostic Products *George Blatt*   7

       Chapter 2   The Role of CDC in Technology Transfer *Dwight
R. Stickney*   11

       Chapter 3   Training and Regulatory Functions of a State
Public Health Laboratory *William J.
Hausler, Jr.*   15

Section II   Systems for the Detection and Identification of
Microorganisms

    Introduction *George W. Campbell*   25

       Chapter 4   Rapid Systems for the Detection of Bacteria
and/or Their Products from Clinical Specimens
William J. Martin   29

Chapter 5   Biochemical "Rapid Identification" of
             Enterobacteriaceae *Henry D. Isenberg*   41

Chapter 6   Immunofluorescence Tests for Bacteria *William
             B. Cherry*   51

Chapter 7   Systems for the Isolation and Identification of
             Anaerobic Bacteria *Genevieve S. Nygaard*   67

Section III   Systems for Clinical Laboratory Immunology

Introduction *Chester M. Zmijewski*   85

Chapter 8   Immunological Diagnosis of Bacterial and Fungal
             Diseases *Dan F. Palmer*   87

Chapter 9   Rapid Diagnosis of Viral Infections *Stanley A.
             Plotkin*   99

Chapter 10   Laboratory Diagnosis of Infectious
             Mononucleosis: Epstein-Barr Virus and the
             Heterophil Test *Jean H. Joncas*   105

Chapter 11   Laboratory Diagnosis of the Autoimmune
             Diseases *Noel R. Rose*   127

Section IV   New Trends in Methodology in Laboratory Microbiology

Introduction *Kenneth R. Cundy*   145

Chapter 12   Radioimmunoassay as Applied to Microbiology
             Martin Fleisher   147

Chapter 13   Radiometric Techniques in Microbiology *Eileen
             L. Randall*   153

Chapter 14   The Use of Gas Chromatography for the
             Identification of Microorganisms *Robert J.
             Mandle and Thomas J. Wade*   163

Chapter 15   The Role of the Computer in Microbiology
*Lawrence J. Kunz, James W. Poitras, Jane
Kissling, Bettie A. Mercier, Marion Cameron,
Carl Lazarus, Robert C. Moellering, Jr., and G.
Octo Barnett*   181

Summary of the Conference   *Vern Pidcoe*   195

Index   199

Participants

Carl Abramson, Ph.D.
Director of Basic Sciences
Pennsylvania College of Podiatric
  Medicine
Philadelphia, Pennsylvania

G. Octo Barnett
Harvard Medical School
Boston, Massachusetts

Josephine T. Bartola, M.Ed., J.D.
Assistant Director
Division of Licensing and Training
Bureau of Laboratories
Pennsylvania Department of Health
Philadelphia, Pennsylvania

George Blatt
Consumer Safety Officer
Division of Diagnostic Product
  Standards and Research
Food and Drug Administration
Rockville, Maryland

Marion Cameron
Harvard Medical School
Boston, Massachusetts

George Campbell, Ph.D.
Chief, Department of Microbiology
Abington Memorial Hospital
Abington, Pennsylvania

William B. Cherry, Ph.D.
Chief, Analytical Bacteriology
  Branch
Bureau of Laboratories
Center for Disease Control
Atlanta, Georgia

Kenneth R. Cundy, Ph.D.
Associate Professor and Director of
  Clinical Microbiology Laboratory
Temple University Health Sciences
  Center
Philadelphia, Pennsylvania

Martin Fleisher, Ph.D.
Memorial Sloan-Kettering Cancer
  Center
New York, New York

Herman Friedman, Ph.D.
Director of Bacteriology
Albert Einstein Medical Center, and
Professor of Microbiology
Temple University Health Sciences
  Center
Philadelphia, Pennsylvania

William J. Hausler, Jr., Ph.D.
Director, State Hygienic Laboratory
University of Iowa
Iowa City, Iowa

Henry D. Isenberg, Ph.D.
Attending Microbiologist, and
Professor of Clinical Pathology
Long Island Jewish-Hillside Medical
  Center
New Hyde Park, New York

Jean H. Joncas, M.D.
Director of Infectious Diseases
Ste. Justine Hospital of the Univer-
  sity of Montreal, and
Research Associate
The Institute of Microbiology of
  Montreal
Montreal, Quebec, Canada

Jane Kissling
Harvard Medical School
Boston, Massachusetts

Lawrence J. Kunz, Ph.D.
Bacteriology Laboratories
Massachusetts General Hospital
Boston, Massachusetts

Carl Lazarus
Harvard Medical School
Boston, Massachusetts

Robert J. Mandle, Ph.D.
Professor of Microbiology
Thomas Jefferson University
Philadelphia, Pennsylvania

William J. Martin, Ph.D.
Chief, Microbiology Section
Clinical Laboratories
University of California at Los
  Angeles Hospital and Clinics, and
Adjunct Associate Professor of
  Pathology and Immunology
School of Medicine, University of
  California
Los Angeles, California

Bettie A. Mercier
Harvard Medical School
Boston, Massachusetts

Robert C. Moellering, Jr.
Harvard Medical School
Boston, Massachusetts

Genevieve S. Nygaard
Supervisor, Special Bacteriology
Microbial Diseases Laboratory
California Department of Health
Berkeley, California

Dan F. Palmer, Dr. P.H.
Bureau of Laboratories
Center for Disease Control
Atlanta, Georgia

Vern Pidcoe, Dr. P.H.
Assistant Director
Bureau of Laboratories
Pennsylvania Department of Health,
  and
Adjunct Associate Professor of
  Microbiology
Temple University Health Sciences
  Center
Philadelphia, Pennsylvania

Stanley A. Plotkin, M.D.
Children's Hospital of Philadelphia,
  and
The Wistar Institute of Anatomy and
  Biology
Philadelphia, Pennsylvania

James W. Poitras
Harvard Medical School
Boston, Massachusetts

James E. Prier, D.V.M., Ph.D.
Director, Bureau of Laboratories
Pennsylvania Department of Health,
    and
Adjunct Professor of Microbiology
Temple University Health Sciences
    Center
Philadelphia, Pennsylvania

Eileen L. Randall, Ph.D.
Clinical Microbiologist
Department of Pathology and
    Laboratory Medicine
Evanston Hospital
Evanston, Illinois, and
Associate Professor of Clinical
    Pathology
Northwestern University Medical
    Center
Chicago, Illinois

Noel R. Rose, M.D., Ph.D.
Chairman, Department of
    Immunology and Microbiology
Wayne State University
Detroit, Michigan

Jay E. Satz, Ph.D.
Director, Division of Virology and
    Immunology
Bureau of Laboratories
Pennsylvania Department of Health
Philadelphia, Pennsylvania

John C. Sherris, M.D.
Professor and Chairman
Department of Microbiology
University of Washington
Seattle, Washington

Dwight R. Stickney, M.D.
Assistant to the Director
Bureau of Laboratories
Center for Disease Control
Atlanta, Georgia

Chester Zmijewski, Ph.D.
Director, Tissue Typing Laboratory
The William Pepper Laboratory
Hospital of the University of
    Pennsylvania
Philadelphia, Pennsylvania

Recent and Future Changes in the Clinical Microbiology Laboratory

John C. Sherris

Until 10 or 15 years ago, the only major changes in methodological principles and in the operation of the average clinical microbiology laboratory since the 1920's were the addition of some tests associated with developments in chemotherapy. There had been dramatic changes in diagnostic virology with the introduction of tissue culture techniques, of course, but these applications were generally limited to some larger public health laboratories. Clinical microbiology in most institutions tended to be highly individualistic, favorite and unique procedures abounded, and experience often carried more weight than objectivity. Concepts of quality control, proficiency evaluation, and methodological standardization were seldom applied and were often regarded with suspicion. Training was frequently quite unstructured and many of those performing clinical microbiological procedures in smaller institutions had few qualifications for the task. Many of us in the field at that time looked with some embarrassment at the developments in technology and performance control which were occurring in clinical chemistry, but consoled ourselves with the thought that our own discipline was much more difficult (which it is), required the continuous application of informed judgment (which it does), and was, therefore, perhaps, inappropriate for the application of statistical standards of performance and the use of automated procedures (which it is not). It was with a sense of considerable shock that we learned from the studies of Dr. Morris Schaeffer and his colleagues (1) just how poor the standards of performance were in many clinical laboratories, and I believe that this was a turning point toward a resurgence of interest in clinical microbiology and the improvement in its practice which has taken place in the past few years.

In the symposium which follows, many of the most important recent technical advances in the field will be covered, as will new and important developments in regulation and training. Therefore, I will address myself mainly to some other areas of advance and change that I believe to be very important, and then will try to look briefly into the future.

There have been several recent important technical developments in the subject, and more may be anticipated at an accelerating rate. Some of these have been concerned with the simplification of existing procedures to make them more readily available to the average laboratory. Under this heading can be considered a variety of kits which permit the easy application of multiple substrate tests and which depend on the extensive use of plastics. Also, kits for a variety of serological tests and spot test methods for rapid biochemical procedures have come into wide use. Each of these procedures has required, or needs, extensive comparative testing with traditional methods to insure an adequate level of accuracy and reproducibility. New methods for detecting early microbial growth and microbial antigens in situ have been developed. New and more sensitive serological techniques have come into use both for detecting immune responses to a variety of microbial pathogens and for demonstrating free antigen in blood or in cerebrospinal fluid, and it seems certain that counter immunoelectrophoretic techniques will play an increasing role in the work of the clinical microbiology laboratory in the future. Technical developments have led to a much greater understanding of infections due to anaerobic organisms and have facilitated their diagnosis and identification. In particular, the introduction of gas chromatography as a diagnostic and identification procedure has simplified, speeded, and improved identification methods. I will not attempt to list all the new technical developments which have occurred, but the above will serve as important examples.

In addition to technical developments, there has been a growing acceptance of the need for methodological standardization of procedures whose results are themselves method dependent. The recognition of this need was first apparent in the case of serological tests for syphilis, and great benefits have resulted from the application of the standardized procedures developed in the Venereal Diseases Research Laboratory. Antimicrobic susceptibility testing is another example where methodological standardization promises to eliminate many of the confusions of the past. The acceptance by the Food and Drug Administration (FDA) (2, 3) and tentatively by the National Committee for Clinical Laboratory Standards (NCCLS) of the same basic diffusion procedure can be expected to yield better interlaboratory repro-

ducibility and a better base line for studies with both new and old anti-microbics in the future. There is need for extension of this approach, particularly to serodiagnostic tests for disease other than syphilis, because the absence of standard or reference procedures continues to encourage much individuality which is often reflected in an inability to relate quantitative data derived in different laboratories. Standardized procedures must be reviewed from time to time and up-dated when new technological or procedural developments render the old ones obsolete. This is best handled by a formal annual or biennial review.

Quality control procedures have now become a routine in most laboratories and are required for those subject to the federal Clinical Laboratories Improvement Act (CLIA). Excellent guides to the application of quality control procedures have been published (4, 5) and the only word of caution needed is that they should not be "overcomplexified" and divert so much of a laboratory's resources that attention to the work itself is impaired. It is to be hoped that performance standards for many commercial media and reagents will become widely adopted and that quality control data on these will be made available by the manufacturers to the individual user so that their own quality assurance programs can be developed on the basis of this knowledge.

Acceptance of both voluntary and mandatory proficiency testing during the past few years has been dramatic and has certainly had beneficial effects on performance, and special credit should be given to the College of American Pathologists for pioneering this approach. Hopefully, by now, almost every laboratory is enrolled in one such proficiency testing scheme. The major function of proficiency testing should be educational because the great majority of laboratories and laboratory workers wish to improve their performance. All evaluation tests should be followed up by a complete analysis of results, the reasons for errors, and recommended procedures for correcting them. Excessive emphasis on regulatory aspects of proficiency testing may be self-defeating by focusing efforts on how to get an acceptable answer to a particular test specimen rather than on how to improve overall quality.

Another development which may certainly be expected to improve standards in clinical microbiology is the wider adoption of registration and certification examinations as a means to identify qualified individuals at various levels of responsibility. The American Board of Medical Microbiology and the National Registry of Microbiologists under the auspices of the American Academy of Microbiology have greatly extended the opportunities in this regard, and their diplomates have now been recognized in a number of federal and state laws and regulations. Hopefully, all those who are qualified but who have not obtained certification or registration by these or other appropriate bodies, such as the American Board of Pathology or the Registry of Medical Technologists of the American Society for Clinical Pathology

(ASCP), will do so, because this increases the ability of the certifying organizations to meet their primary objective of improved standards of performance.

Training in clinical microbiology, particularly at the postdoctoral level, has improved considerably · during the past 15 years. Programs were encouraged by the American Academy of Microbiology and several were supported by the National Institutes of Health (NIH). Unfortunately, this source of support has now almost ceased, but several institutions have managed to obtain residency positions specifically for training Ph.D. and M.D. clinical microbiologists. Probably 100 or so clinical microbiologists have passed through these programs into positions of responsibility, and have, in turn, extended training opportunities to others at all levels. At approximately the same time, opportunities for spending up to 2 years training in clinical microbiology have been incorporated in some clinical pathology residencies, and this too is contributing to the pool of well-trained individuals. To supplement these developments, a number of new M.S. programs in clinical or medical microbiology have been developed specifically to provide additional training and education for those who seek technical supervisory positions. These are particularly important programs because the technical supervision has been shown to be the key to good laboratory performance. Hopefully, federal granting agencies will recognize the need for continued support of these programs and there will be some restitution of funds that have been cut off.

There have been great advances in continuing education in clinical microbiology in recent years, as exemplified by this program. The ASCP has been providing a series of workshops and manuals staffed and written by their own members and many by other leading microbiologists. These have been generally excellent. More recently, the Board of Education and Training of the American Society for Microbiology (ASM) has initiated workshops and regional conferences and they too have been highly successful. ASM branches have developed strong clinical sections, and many smaller regional clinical and public health microbiological societies have sprung up in response to the heightened interest in the subject.

Finally, means of scientific communication in the field are improving dramatically. The new ASM *Manual of Clinical Microbiology* (4) is now being supplemented by the ASM *Cumitechs* (6) to provide continuing and up-to-date information and recommendations on technical methods and laboratory procedures. Excellent workshop manuals have been produced by the ASCP Council on Microbiology and many good monographs have recently appeared. In addition, the clinical microbiologists will now have their own *Journal of Clinical Microbiology* through the ASM Publications Office.

Thus, the past few years have been a period of great advance, although much yet remains to be done to improve the quality of work for our patients. At the very least, the framework for a highly effective clinical microbiological service has been developed and further improvements can be expected.

One area of microbiology in which change has been slow to come about on any large scale has been in that of automation and mechanization. Many procedures which are obvious candidates for mechanization are still performed manually, and the time spent in repetitive routine work often deviates effort from the more complicated microbiological problems that can only be resolved by the trained microbiologist. For example, machines for spreading plates under controlled atmospheric conditions are still not available; staining machines are used little; equipment for monitoring growth and for automatic subculture to multiple substrates at night are entirely feasible and test results could be read out automatically. Only now is antimicrobic susceptibility testing being automated and are computers being adapted to information storage and retrieval and quality control in microbiology. The delay in the application of available technology is partly because manufacturers have underestimated the market potential and this, in turn, is partly due to an inherent conservatism among clinical microbiologists which is reflected in a negative response to market surveys for new developments. There is, I believe, little doubt that new developments of this type will become increasingly available and will rapidly find their place in the average laboratory.

Looking further into the future, we can expect more sophisticated and totally new approaches to be adopted in clinical microbiology. For example, the automated measurement of a variety of physicochemical characteristics of microorganisms and their analysis by computer pattern recognition systems seems a likely possibility for rapid identification. Such an approach will probably require the development of new taxonomic criteria and the development of better defined media. Even more sensitive detection or microbial growth and indirect optical methods for quantitation can be anticipated. Susceptibility testing may be at the cellular level and assays will become increasingly specific and accurate through enzymic or radioimmunological techniques. The overall objectives will be toward increasing accuracy and precision and more rapid results, especially for situations of clinical urgency.

It will be very important, as new technical developments are introduced, that we bear in mind continually the ultimate purpose of clinical microbiology which is to develop the means for providing the optimal data required for patient care as reliably and economically as possible and as rapidly as can be achieved in cases of clinical urgency. We should recognize the risk that the production of redundant data may obscure rather than illuminate, and that seeking levels of precision which are clinically irrelevant may enhance costs without value to the patient or the science. The application of judgment, based on knowledge and experience to clinical microbiological work and its interpretation, will continue to remain critical to good performance, and automated systems will extend the capability rather than replace the clinical microbiologist.

Even closer cooperation between the clinical microbiologist and the clinician will be needed in the future as the proportion of immunologically compromised patients and of opportunistic infections continues to increase. Greater attention to the quality of specimens and to using all available procedures to assess the pathogenic role of organisms in mixed culture will be needed. Rapid diagnosis of opportunistic viral and fungal infections will become more important and in vitro assessment of the effects of combined chemotherapeutics will be more commonly needed. Environmental and epidemiological aspects of microbiology will become an even more important aspect of the work of the clinical microbiologist, and all of this will be facilitated by newer technical developments.

A final word about a neglected area of research—I believe that further effort should be put into evaluations of the effectiveness of the numerous variations in microbiological routines that are employed and of the use to which clinical microbiological data is put in patient care. The results of such studies can guide us as to the most valuable and efficient use of our resources and can help to remove one of the last major areas of subjectivity and contention from the discipline.

LITERATURE CITED

1. Schaeffer, M., D. Widelock, S. Blatt, and M. E. Wilson. 1967. The clinical laboratory improvement program in New York City. I. Methods of evaluation and results of performance tests. Health Lab. Sci. 4:72–89.
2. Rules and regulations. 1972. Antibiotic susceptibility discs. Federal Register 37:20525–20529.
3. Rules and regulations. 1973. Antibiotic susceptibility discs—correction. Federal Register 38:2576.
4. Lennette, E. H., E. H. Spaulding, and J. P. Truant. 1974. Manual of clinical microbiology. American Society for Microbiology, Washington, D.C.
5. Bartlett, R. C., W. R. Irving, Jr., and C. Rutz. 1968. Quality control in clinical microbiology. American Society of Clinical Pathologists Commission on Continuing Education, Chicago, Ill.
6. Bartlett, R. C., P. D. Ellner, and J. A. Washington II. 1974. Blood cultures. Cumitech #1. J. C. Sherris (ed. coord.), American Society for Microbiology, Washington, D. C.

SECTION I

The Increased Role of Regulatory Agencies in Microbiology

Introduction

During the past decade there have been at least four distinct events which have significantly affected the characteristics of the practice of clinical microbiology. They are: (a) the requirement that purveyors of medical services to Social Security recipients meet specified standards, including quality of performance; (b) the enactment of the CLIA 1967; (c) the development of state regulations in a number of jurisdictions for the purpose of setting standards of performance; and (d) the recent decision by the FDA to extend its regulatory influences into the field of in vitro diagnostics.

None of these new regulatory activities developed without controversy. States have challenged the assumed prerogatives of federal agencies, private interests have jousted with state officials, and arguments have been conducted within agencies. And as each step of each program has been implemented, it has been fraught with controversy, regardless of the jurisdiction involved. Viewed in retrospect, for the most part such antagonisms have been highly productive. They have not existed for the purpose of destroying proposals, but rather to assure that a result of optimal public benefit will be achieved. In other words, they have been, and continue to be, part of a great debate which is a medley of challenges to authority, criticisms of objectives, and playing of the devil's advocate. Because of it all, regulatory programs in the field of clinical laboratory medicine have developed with a perspective that may be unique among government control measures of public and private services.

3

My own experience, and that of most state laboratory directors, has been with the problems of local regulatory programs as they are correlated with Medicare requirements, and also with the provisions of the CLIA 1967 as they affect individual laboratory operations within the states. On a more philosophical level, state laboratory directors have engaged in a continuing discourse with federal agencies on the proper provisions, objectives, and characteristics of an optimal long-term laboratory regulatory program. This dialogue occurs most frequently with members of the Center for Disease Control (CDC). For the casual observer of a session involving CDC members and state laboratory directors, it might appear that a great antagonism exists. In reality, the traditional controversy is by design, and has proved to be one of the most productive methods available to achieve an appropriate result in matters of primary concern to both federal and state agencies.

There has been less experience between state laboratory regulatory officers and the FDA. Already a number of groups, notably those representing industry, have expressed discontent with the concept of regulating in vitro reagents. Some of this relates to the apprehension normally associated with any new and somewhat unknown regulatory program. For the most part, state agencies have not demonstrated a strong influence in this area, and have accepted the attitude of cautious observation. I have had some occasion to discuss this area with FDA officials, and have the impression that there is already a good basis for assuming that a productive dialogue will be developing among the concerned agencies.

Certainly there has been a central theme common to the various regulatory programs which have been developed over the past 10 years. This is, in summary, that a primary and over-riding objective is to improve the performance of clinical laboratory services. Although such an objective is inherent in regulations in other fields, it is unusual that a concentrated effort by the regulatory agencies is effected to offer the mechanism to achieve the objective. It is not coincidental, for example, the CLIA has the word "Improvement" in the title.

In both federal and state jurisdictions the licensee is not left alone to seek out the road to compliance. A wide variety of training programs for personnel, consulting aids, and other mechanisms are used. Even proficiency evaluations are more frequently used as a method for detecting and correcting deficiencies than as a policing tool. There is, perhaps, some current concern that this approach to regulation will not continue in the future, but its real value from the standpoint of public benefit seems to be apparent.

There may be a tendency to assume that the establishment and enforcement of regulations is a rather simple straightforward procedure. A review of advisory committee meetings, *Federal Register* details, and journal reports indicates that simplicity is not a characteristic of regulation design and enforcement. Representatives of both CDC and FDA can testify to the amount of discussion, testimony, and changes that accompany any proposed regulation. And, to a lesser degree, the same complexities confuse and complicate regulation development at the state level. Establishment of statutory authorities, of course, is even more complicating, requiring the joint efforts of scientists, politicians, journalists, government and private industry employees, and generally as strange and curious a group of bedfellows as can be imagined.

CHAPTER 1

Food and Drug Administration Regulation of in Vitro Diagnostic Products

George Blatt

In January 1972, FDA published a notice in the *Federal Register* indicating its intent to begin an active program to regulate in vitro diagnostic products. This announcement caused a rather large ripple of concern in the industry which we intended to regulate—this was to be anticipated.

The program was initiated as a result of disturbing information from several sources. Individual concerned laboratory scientists had begun to question the erratic or poor quality of commercially available diagnostic products, and had done some systematic studies which were reported in the literature. These results were alarming. Simultaneously, the FDA began to receive an increasing number of complaints from individual laboratory professionals, indicating a widespread problem. Eventually, we sponsored some limited studies of widely used diagnostic products to obtain some information based on controlled studies. The results generally supported the earlier reported work.

The labeling inadequacies might have been amusing had the potential consequences not been so frightening. We saw labeling procedures which experienced laboratory scientists could not follow. We even saw instructions which would have required the operator to have three hands. These observations suggested that industry was not policing itself adequately. The reaction of the professional users of these vital clinical laboratory products surprised and, eventually, concerned us. This reaction primarily took the form of silence or expressions of concern that the federal government was about to interfere in the professional practice of clinical science and medicine. Needless to say, such concerns were unfounded.

In 1972, the total headquarters personnel commitment to this program was three persons. In the intervening 2¾ years, the agency has made substantial commitments to the intentions stated in that original announcement. During this period, the original Diagnostic Products Staff, currently the Division of Diagnostic Product Standards and Research, was incorporated into the new Bureau of Medical Devices and Diagnostic Products, with a concomitant increase in staff and support resources.

In August 1972, the agency published in the *Federal Register* a broad proposal of the regulatory scheme by which it intended to regulate these products. At the basis of this scheme were two major activities: the establishment of a uniform labeling format for all in vitro diagnostic products and the establishment of product class standards for various groups of products intended for similar or related uses. In March 1973, the final order of these regulations was established with an effective date of September 1974 for compliance with the labeling provisions of the regulation.

Even before the effective date for compliance with the labeling regulations, substantial and beneficial changes in the total spectrum of in vitro diagnostic product labeling occurred. This took the form of more adequate disclosure of product composition, instructions for users, and proper presentation of test results.

The labeling for every product should now be in compliance with the labeling regulations. We are not so naive as to believe this is the case, but there is reason to consider that most of the products that are being shipped are properly labeled. However, as a regulatory agency we have an obligation to assure compliance, and cannot trust to the good will and high intentions of the regulated industry.

Toward this end, a program is being instituted which will result in each manufacturer of these products being visited at least once during the next 2 years. These visits will be primarily for the purpose of determining compliance with the labeling requirements of the regulations, but will also, in many cases, extend to inspection of production facilities and control systems. It is our intention to identify not only the apparent weaknesses in individual manufacturing plants, but also to identify those elements of manufacture and control which represent an acceptable level of manufacturing control.

Under legislation now pending before Congress, the FDA will have a statutory responsibility to promulgate "good manufacturing practices" regulations which will be binding on all manufacturers of these products. We hope to be well along toward this goal at the passage of this legislation.

The development of product class standards appears to represent more of a concern to professional users. In some way, this activity was interpreted as a move by the government to standardize the methodologies on which diagnostic products were based and thereby reduce the number of available products. Nothing could be further from the truth. Product class standards, as they are developed, will essentially be statements of acceptable performance limits for groups of products. These limits will be useful and reasonable.

The standards development procedure, which is clearly set out in the regulation, allows for submission of data and information and relevant comment of any sort from any interested party. Procedurally, the first step is a "call for data and information" to determine the need for a standard. Our first call for data and information was issued in May 1973 for products intended for the measurement or detection of glucose or total sugars. The information received in response to that call indicated the need for a product class standard. Subsequently, we issued a proposed glucose product class standard in the *Federal Register,* which also invited comments from all interested parties. The closing date for comment on that proposed product class standard was December 12, 1974.

In November 1973, a call was published for calibrators used in clinical chemistry procedures and in March 1974, for products used for the measurement of hemoglobin. Proposed standards for these groups have not yet been published.

Perhaps of equal interest to microbiologists and of more direct relevance, is that the next three calls for data and information for the development of standards are in the microbiological area: products intended for nontreponemal tests for syphilis, rabies, and rubella.

One of the aspects of this program which has been most productive has been the continuing communication between the agency, manufacturers, trade associations, and the significant input of our scientific advisers. This latter input has taken the form of active cooperation between the FDA and the Center for Disease Control (CDC) as well as exceptional assistance provided to the program by our scientific advisory committee. The development of a successful program from the perspective of the patient depends upon an open expression of opinions from various perspectives.

I did not mention professional associations as having provided significant positive input. With few exceptions, the professional societies and associations have remained silent during the development of this program which has a critical impact on their very livelihood and their professional activities. In fairness, I must say that the situation has improved somewhat since the inception of the program. Professional scientific societies such as the American Society for Microbiology represent not only a highly expert body of scientific knowledge but also a group which is intimately knowledgeable about products in use and, therefore, the advantages and disadvantages of various products and methodologies. The purpose of the FDA program is simply to improve the quality of products and, therefore, the quality of results. I am sure that any comments from professional organizations will receive full and adequate consideration.

What is the basis for the lack of active participation by the laboratory professional? We in the government have a limited view of the "real world" of laboratory science. On an individual basis, many laboratory scientists have expressed a fatalistic acceptance of big government enveloping their lives. I find that regrettable. We look to laboratory professionals as partners in this venture and value their opinions. Programs such as this are not inexorable, unchangeable, or inflexible. We have heard the complaint of government interference in medicine or science many times. However, we see our role simply to assist and protect the patient, by assuring that those who deliver direct health services have the most reliable and accurate tools with which to work.

You have heard me refer to our "call for data and information" as a mechanism for determining the need for a product class standard. I spoke of the next step, which is a proposed product class standard. There is ample opportunity for you to speak during all phases of our standards development process. We have provided a means by which any party may request the establishment, amendment, or repeal of a product class standard. If these formal mechanisms are too burdensome, write a letter to us. One does not have to make a "federal case" to catch our attention and I believe that we can be responsive to comments, opinions, suggestions, and criticism.

CHAPTER 2

The Role of CDC in Technology Transfer

Clinical laboratory improvement has long been a major program for the CDC's Bureau of Laboratories. This program is multifaceted, consisting of development of technology through basic and applied research, improvement in mechanisms for transfer of technology, direct analytical services offered at CDC, biological product evaluation, and standardization of biological products. The laboratory is of central importance to the effectiveness of all health activities—clinical, public, and investigative. Furthermore, it is our belief that the quality and efficiency of health laboratories, whenever and however improved, will result in better quality and more effective health care delivery.

Regulation of clinical laboratories is relatively new. The Congress of the United States passed the Clinical Laboratory Improvement Act in 1967. This action was necessary for several reasons, and, of these, three were of major concern. First, laboratory test results are often inaccurate. Today, marginal or erroneous health laboratory performance may consume as much as 2% of the gross national product in direct and indirect costs to the health care system and to the patient. Second, the cost to the consumer for laboratory services is increasing; in essence, the nation's laboratories are a multibillion dollar industry. The Stanford Research Institute recently found that the average cost per test in 1968 was $3.50 to $4.00, and, in 1972, $3.00 to $3.50. Furthermore, the average cost per test in 1975 is expected to be $2.75 (1). The number of tests performed annually has increased from 0.8 billion in

11

1964 to 4 billion in 1974 and is expected to exceed 6.6 billion in 1980. Therefore, dollar volume is expected to rise over the next 5 years from $11 billion to over $16.5 billion in 1980 (2). In a recent study by the Investment Research Department of the First National New York City Bank (2), it was found that the growth rate of laboratory tests in the past decade averaged 17%/year, and, in 1975, a base growth rate of at least 10–12% will be established. The growth rate is expected to increase to 18% or more during the mid-1970's as a result of an increase in employee/employer prepaid health insurance plans, the enactment of more comprehensive national health care legislation, and greater use of preventive medicine techniques. The third concern, and a very important one, is the potential for unnecessary human suffering as a result of inaccurate laboratory test results. To quote Dr. Raymond Gambino (3) of Columbia Presbyterian Medical Center, "Lab tests have become more important in detecting many diseases than the physical examination. It is now an extension of the physical exam."

For the reasons mentioned above, the Bureau of Laboratories of the Center for Disease Control is concerned with how well laboratory tests are performed.

The CDC was granted administrative authority for the CLIA in 1967. Basically, the act sets minimum standards of good laboratory practice in the four general areas of personnel, quality control, facilities and equipment, and performance. Although the CLIA is applicable to only a small number of the nation's clinical laboratories, we regard it as a model program designed to insure clinical laboratory services of uniform high quality. This does not mean that we feel our program is the only possible model or that it does not have shortcomings. We have, however, learned a great deal in the short history of the program and our objective is not only to improve the proficiency of clinical laboratories, as the name of the act implies, but also to improve our own capabilities in administering the program.

The implementation of this program was a vast undertaking; standards are not easily developed. Consequently, the CDC sought and still seeks additional help in the form of advice from "experts" serving on ad hoc advisory panels in specific areas of laboratory science. After working with these groups, the scientists prepare a document covering a particular area and submit it to the state health laboratory directors for review and comment. Their suggestions are then included in the document as appropriate. Additional review is made by the CDC Medical Laboratory Services Advisory Committee, the members of which are knowledgeable in specialized areas of laboratory sciences and represent a geographical cross-section of the country. Finally, the document is published in the *Federal Register* for public comment. This process is very time-consuming; however, it is the most efficient way to insure the development of reasonable laboratory standards.

By this process, the qualifications were devised for the laboratory director and supervisors. New ideas about qualifying personnel are centered around the concept of the technologist supervisor, a person with laboratory training at the technician level and subsequent experience in a specified area of laboratory medicine such as bacteriology. This supervisor would be expected to be knowledgable in the discipline and aware of recently published literature in order to make independent judgments at the bench level.

As standards were developed for quality control, checklists were designed to aid in assessing a laboratory's internal quality control, methods, and handling of specimens and reports. More specific checklists will soon be completed which will make possible more objective collection of data for computer analysis. Incorporated into these checklists will be specific questions about the laboratory's facilities and equipment.

Performance evaluation through proficiency testing first took the form of a defined discipline as a result of CLIA 1967. Although for many years CDC had carried out limited proficiency testing activities and the College of American Pathologists had conducted its "quality surveys," the concept of a surveillance system to detect poor laboratory performance and to improve it began with CLIA. Presently, proficiency testing involves test samples being mailed to participating laboratories. Since they are identified as test samples, they are generally handled differently than routine samples. In effect, the measured performance level of the laboratory is the best that can be demonstrated. Presently, other means of assessing laboratory performance are being investigated. These are internal and external blind samples, on-site samples, and patient specimens.

Since the inception of the CLIA, improvement has been demonstrated in licensed laboratories participating for 2 years or more.

The program emphasis is on laboratory improvement, not on regulation. Licensure and proficiency testing is only a small part of the Bureau of Laboratories; however, the information obtained from this activity is used as a guide in directing and coordinating established programs of laboratory training and applied research activities. Future efforts are being directed toward establishment of one set of standards for all clinical laboratories. With the publication of the Medicare independent laboratory regulations, in the *Federal Register* (September 19, 1974) (4), which are in line with the CLIA regulations, this effort has been partially realized. However, many clinical laboratories remain outside the jurisdiction of these regulations. The CDC is making every effort to extend regulations to cover all clinical laboratories. Administering a program that requires all laboratories to use a minimal set of standards is a vast undertaking. This would more than likely be a collaborative program between agencies of the Department of Health, Education, and Welfare and state health departments. The details of such a program have not been worked out; however, state health agencies would be expected to play a major role in the development and administration of such a program.

Another aspect of the CDC program in the transfer of technology is diagnostic product evaluation. The CDC produces and distributes approximately 1,700 microbiological and immunological reference reagents to manufacturers of in vitro diagnostic products, state laboratories, the Pan American

Health Organization (PAHO), and the World Health Organization (WHO). In addition, product specifications and reference methods for approximately 2,000 products have been developed by CDC; these are available to industry for use as the criteria of product acceptability in the formal premarket evaluation program. A list of product lots tested at CDC and found to be satisfactory is distributed monthly to state laboratories, federal agencies, PAHO, WHO, and other interested organizations or individuals. This list, in turn, is often sent by the state laboratories and WHO to clinical laboratories under their jurisdiction. The need for the development of standards for diagnostic products became even more obvious when CDC was given responsibility for administering the CLIA. It was soon noticed that part of the poor performance in the nation's clinical laboratories could be attributed to the products used by laboratories and not to internal operations. At this time CDC proposed a regulatory program for diagnostic products, but it was determined that the FDA already had the authority to administer such a program.

Regardless of where the authority is vested within the federal government, the staff at the CDC has a broad technical capability and many years of experience which is of considerable value to the FDA in developing its regulatory program. Our role in the in vitro diagnostic products program is to supply technical capability to support the FDA's regulatory authority.

An integral part of the laboratory improvement program is training. This is provided through field and headquarters courses, assistance to state public health laboratories in course presentations, and technical consultation. The objective of training is to improve the quality of health laboratory services through more effective laboratory manpower development, performance of technical procedures, and application of managerial skills. The CDC makes every effort to train teachers and/or consultants so that the skills learned can be successively passed on to the largest audience possible. Demand for CDC laboratory procedural manuals and visual aids has increased 4-fold over the last 3 years. New training courses and manuals are developed and made available as soon as new procedures are ready for use in the clinical laboratory. Thus, through training and regulatory surveillance programs, progress is being made toward the goal of laboratory improvement.

LITERATURE CITED

1. Stanford Research Institute World Markets for Nonpharmaceutical Health Products. 1969. Report 383, Oct.
2. The Clinical Laboratory Industry. 1973. A survey by the First National City Bank Investment Research Department, pp. 10–13.
3. Gambino, R. 1970. The commercial lab puzzle. Med. Lab. Observ. May–June, p. 23.
4. Federal Register. 1974. 39: 33,690–33,698.

CHAPTER 3

Training and Regulatory Functions of a State Public Health Laboratory

William J. Hausler, Jr.

Many of you know Iowa by having flown over the state on your way to the west coast or by passing through on Interstate 80 which traverses the state. On the other hand, many of you think you know Iowa but get it confused with Idaho or, yes, even sometimes with Ohio. You know it is out west somewhere but are just not exactly sure. To refresh your geography, it lies between the Mississippi River on the east and the Missouri River on the west and is between Minnesota and Missouri on the north and south. Our laboratories are located in the southeast quarter of the state in Iowa City. Mr. John M. Cheever wrote a very descriptive article of the peace and tranquility of our community as well as our state (1). Many of us are careful though not to encourage too many people to absorb this atmosphere because we do not want it to become overpopulated. In his attempt to move people on, John Cheever wrote, "If you like it here, you will love Omaha."

These introductory remarks are not intended to make this a Chamber of Commerce presentation about the state of Iowa, the University of Iowa, or, for that matter Iowa City. However, I hope to draw your attention in the next few minutes to our attitudes on training and regulatory functions of state public health laboratories in contrast to what I view as the attitudes of the other states. Our relaxed mode of life, our protection of basic individual freedoms, and our attitudes toward one another all bear on the main issue of our discussion.

15

When all of the state laboratories are lumped together and discussed as a group, we sometimes fail to recognize their individuality or uniqueness. But consider these factors for a moment. Each state laboratory is governed by an administrative channel unique to that particular state. The director of the laboratory may report directly to the head of the health department, to another division chief, to two or more agency administrators, or, as in our case, directly to the President of the University. These administrative channels greatly affect the manner in which programs are conceived, developed, and moved forward to action. Some do so with considerable ease and others with extreme difficulties.

We must also recognize the innate qualities of the laboratory director. The attitude of the director concerning his own activities in administration, agency or governmental politics, and personal goals and desires for achievement all have a bearing upon the programs and policies of the laboratory. As I said earlier, to lump state laboratories together and discuss them in one program context is nearly impossible. On any subject of your choosing the 50 laboratories will display themselves in almost a normal curve. Admittedly, on some issues or subjects, such as syphilis serology, the range will be very narrow, whereas on others, such as training and regulation, the range will be broad.

In order for me to present to you what other state laboratories are doing in training and regulatory functions, I feel it is necessary to explain what we are doing and not doing in Iowa. Then I would like to contrast these programs with those of other states of whom I really have only limited knowledge.

Because the Iowa laboratory has always been a part of an educational institution, its leadership and staff have been more prone to the development of educational programs of a variety of types. In this same context, regulatory attitudes, philosophies, or programs are not a part of our activities and we have little initiative in this regard.

Our prime focus is to have available a staff with broad professional interests who can provide the state of Iowa with the highest caliber of service. In addition to their appointment in the laboratory, a number of our staff also hold appointments in the College of Medicine and/or the College of Dentistry. These are full academic appointments and not of the adjunct type. These individuals present courses, team-teach in other courses, guide graduate student programs, or otherwise advise and counsel graduate and professional students.

The net effect of these dual appointments and working in an academic atmosphere is an awareness of meeting educational needs through a variety of modes. Educational efforts are not directed solely to the various health laboratories and their component staffs. The continuing education efforts of the Colleges of Medicine, Dentistry, and Nursing, as well as the School of

Pharmacy, provide appropriate outlets for our own educational efforts. It is our opinion that all segments of the health professional community need to be informed of advances in laboratory science and technology—not just the laboratory worker.

Although educational contacts are made through formal college credit courses and continuing education courses for other groups, we also conduct our own program. Many aspects to this important phase of our operations are intertwined for a total effort.

For a number of years, our laboratories presented one, two, or maybe three laboratory training courses annually in bacteriology, serology, parasitology, and water and wastewater sanitation. In addition, the laboratory was constantly used for bench training in a variety of specialized techniques. The state laboratory resource was being utilized, but not to its potential.

Then, about a decade ago, we all experienced the beginning of revolutionary rather than evolutionary changes in laboratory programs and in support of other programs. We experienced the introduction of Medicare and the rules and regulations applicable to hospital and independent laboratories. Following this event was the enactment of the CLIA which regulates interstate laboratories and then a passel of related activities such as state licensure and/or regulation, manpower development, clinical laboratory standards, regulation of diagnostic products and many more. Recently new federal laws in occupational health and safety as well as environmental control programs in air, water, wastewater, and radiological health have emerged. To meet these many new challenges in laws and regulations, state laboratories have been forced to redefine their roles in order to meet these challenges.

In Iowa, a voluntary laboratory improvement program has been developed which is designed to assist the user of laboratory services as well as the provider of these services. A newsletter has also been developed which serves as a "hotline" of information providing the reader with data on the availability of training programs, current disease or health problems, publications of interest, as well as some information on the productive efforts of the state laboratory. The first few issues were distributed only to those laboratories in the syphilis serology appraisal program, but distribution rapidly increased to the current circulation of over 650/issue to persons throughout Iowa, the United States, and internationally. Considering the benefits received, the cost of this publication is extremely low, approximately $100/month.

A performance evaluation program was instituted, as was a rather aggressive continuing education program in the form of workshops, seminars, and field courses. The performance evaluation program covers syphilis and nonsyphilis serology, bacteriology, parasitology, and clinical chemistry. Shipment of unknowns in each category is scheduled 1 year in advance and is published monthly in *Lab Hotline*. As soon as all participant reports are received from a particular shipment, a report is prepared and sent to each participating laboratory. This report contains an analysis of all reported values, their ranges according to the method used, and commentary on the methods of improvement. Again, this program is voluntary and costs the participant nothing.

Information gained from the performance evaluation program is used to design the type of workshops and seminars needed. We build our training program around the deficiencies noted. However, not all training is designed to improve deficiencies. There is also a training advisory committee made up of pathologists and technicians who meet periodically in a retreat setting to discuss and plan new course offerings. All courses are announced well in advance in *Lab Hotline* and are usually scheduled 1 year in advance. This allows those planning to attend to set up their own schedules. The topics covered run the gamut of clinical laboratory activity. Workshops in hematology, enteric bacteriology, enzyme chemistry, parasitology, small hospital bacteriology, laboratory personnel health and safety, and quality control are just a few of the subjects presented.

Other somewhat unique features of the training program include field courses and the accumulation of continuing education units (CEU). Field courses are offered in community colleges, private colleges, or motel facilities. Based upon our experience, we feel that it is easier to take the topic to remote locations rather than to expect those in remote places to expend the time and effort to come to headquarters courses. Topics of field courses are limited only by the availability or ease of transport of necessary equipment and instrumentation. It is obvious that workshops requiring sinks for staining, gas flames, or incubators cannot be presented in motel conference rooms. However, workshops in blood cell morphology and parasitology are easily adapted to these facilities.

Continuing education units are a recent venture of the University of Iowa. Courses are submitted to a university continuing education course evaluator and the number of units are assigned. One CEU is assigned for 10 contact hours. Fractional units are assigned when the course involves less than 10 contact hours. A record is maintained by the university for each individual and, at any given time, he may receive a report of the total number of accumulated CEU's. We feel that this is really a significant new development and will provide the participant with an official record of his endeavors to keep himself currently trained.

Workshops, seminars, and performance evaluation programs are the main vehicles of our educational program, but we have also developed a *Manual of Services* for physicians and health agencies to use in determining those services of the laboratory which will best serve them in any given situation. This also is a most important area of training for state laboratories.

Assistance is provided in training programs conducted by the Iowa Bureau of Labor, on occupational health and safety, for personnel in government agencies and industry, as well as a variety of training programs for those associated with the Iowa Department of Environmental Quality.

One other area which is a form of training, since there are no relative state laws or regulations, is in the evaluation of X-ray and other radiological instrumentation. We evaluate these installations in hospitals that participate in the Medicare program and we also provide the same evaluation service to dentists, chiropractors, or others using these diagnostic tools.

Finally, in discussing training, I should not overlook the benefits achieved by having examiners on our staff who evaluate hospital and independent clinical laboratories under the Medicare program. This service is provided under a contract between our laboratories and the Iowa State Department of Health. During their visits laboratory examiners observe areas where training programs would be worthwhile and also have an opportunity to discuss training needs with a variety of laboratory workers. We are one of many states that would like to assume responsibility for CLIA laboratory review as well, but we have not been successful in getting the CDC to move on our behalf. We feel that we can do a better job of improving performance of all laboratories in our state rather than allowing a few to be examined by the CDC. As a matter of fact, we believe we provide much better service and we have adequate proof for this position.

As can be seen from the foregoing discussion the Iowa program is designed around a voluntary self-help format rather than from a regulatory base. There are no laws governing laboratory operations in Iowa and only these few simple regulations. Each licensed hospital must have minimum laboratory facilities for urinalysis and blood counts. A laboratory performing premarital and prenatal syphilis serologies must be approved by the Iowa State Department of Health and must participate in an appraisal program of the State Hygienic Laboratory.

Several years ago I was an active advocate of the popular belief that the only way to improve laboratory performance was by licensure and/or regulation. I agreed with my colleagues that licensure would weed out the poor and improperly qualified laboratory workers and provide us with a pool of talented individuals upon whom we could depend. I still hold to those basic tenets but not with the same fervor as before. Licensure is a regulatory function that works from the top down, intimidates individuals, and forces them to be reactionary. Licensure also protects the poor performer and provides very limited methods for his removal. True, licensure allows for greater individual mobility but it also allows for the spread of unsatisfactory performance.

I believe that someday we will have some form of licensure in Iowa when the public realizes that it is just as important to protect the public's health by regulation of persons performing critical life-extending analyses as it is to protect them when they have their hair cut, are fitted for a hearing aid or eyeglasses, or when they go to a psychologist or watchmaker. I agree we may be behind the times in this category of involvement but I feel we are far ahead of those who seek licensure legislation first.

Through our various continuing education efforts, we are developing a group of laboratory workers with new and improved diagnostic capabilities. No one is forcing them to seek improvement of their skills, yet we do have evidence of this improvement.

At the beginning of each workshop we give the participants a pretest of the topic or topics to be presented. At the conclusion of the workshop another test is given. Not only do we observe marked improvement in test scores but we also experience an overall improvement in their analysis of proficiency test unknowns in those particular areas. Therefore, we feel that we are improving the skills of laboratorians by these efforts without mandating performance through licensure legislation. If and when licensure does occur in Iowa, the laboratories will already be prepared to a large extent to cope with its restrictive qualities.

These programs are not unique to Iowa, although the manner in which they are presented and operated may be somewhat unique.

As one small aspect of training, let us consider the number of states that provide current information to laboratories through some form of regular publication. As of 1973, 12 out of 50 states published a newsletter with frequency of publication varying from monthly to as needed. Their distribution varies, but primarily they are sent to hospital and other health laboratories. The first laboratory newsletter published with any frequency was that by the Wisconsin State Laboratory of Hygiene beginning in 1961. Iowa came along with its publication in 1965 and 1 or 2 have appeared each year until now there are 12 newsletters of record. It is interesting to note here that I have been contacted by several state laboratory directors who are interested in publishing a newsletter, but invariably their first question concerns the cost of the publication. We are not concerned about cost to any great extent but are more concerned with the educational value achieved.

Another area that seems to be controlled by an unusual attention to cost is laboratory continuing education efforts. I agree that it is a venture with expense but it is not necessary to establish a separate training unit with all of its additional costs. We have a training coordinator whose job it is to develop and schedule workshops and seminars with the instructional staff from our regular laboratory professional staff or outside consultants. All laboratories have some staff slippage that can be utilized in educational endeavors.

In trying to determine the number of states with training programs, I used a 1970 publication of the CDC entitled *Educational Opportunities for Laboratory Personnel* (2). It consists primarily of 492 pages of repetitious data; however, I was able to determine that, as of the date of publication, 23 out of 50 states reportedly provide some form of continuing education. Some of the states limit their efforts to just a few offerings each year in bacteriology and some have active presentations each month on a variety of topics. Again, it is the attitude and dedication of the laboratory administration, as well as the agency location, that appears to determine the frequency and breadth of presentations.

As far as regulatory functions are concerned, the states again differ vastly; however, for purposes of our discussion, we will limit ourselves to those states with laboratory or personnel licensure or regulation. I will summarize the situation as of June 30, 1972. At that time, there were 17 states with a laboratory licensure law, 7 states who only license laboratory personnel, and 5 states with a laboratory registration law. Thus, there are 29 states with laboratory licensure and/or regulation statutes. Elements of each state's licensure statute are as varied as collective training efforts in the state.

What then is the future role of state laboratories? First of all, we must again recall that, when we speak of state laboratories, we must define who they are and what they do. With the rapid development of environmental control programs and occupational health and safety programs, we are witnessing the establishment in some states of new laboratories to support these functions. The classical health department and its laboratory is rapidly changing. At one time it was not difficult to determine who the state laboratory director was—he would be the official delegate in the Association of State and Territorial Public Health Laboratory Directors. Today, in some states, it is difficult to determine who should be the official delegate.

If there is a feeling of frustration in designating the facility in each state that will serve as the official state health laboratory, think of the frustration that each state laboratory experiences in working with federal agencies. Depending on program parameters, state laboratories must work with the CDC, the FDA, the Social Security Administration, the Environmental Protection Agency, and the U. S. Department of Labor, to name just a few. What is really needed is the development of a partnership between federal and state agencies that will clearly establish the prerogatives of each. A case in point is the overlapping and redundancy of laboratory examinations and certification conducted by both the CDC and many states. Federal programs should be designed in a manner to provide for enforcement by each state rather than enforcement by the responsible federal agency. An example is the recently enacted 55 miles/hour speed limit. How foolish it would be to have a federal police force to enforce this law. It is equally absurd to employ federal examiners to enforce laboratory licensure laws when the capability exists in the states. We need uniform regulations, as we have with the 55 miles/hour speed limit and automobile emission control devices, to allow mobility within and between states but enforced by state authorities.

It is my personal opinion that until we have uniform regulations we will continue to invite persons to speak on training and regulatory functions of state public health laboratories and we will continue to be exposed to a chaotic situation. State laboratories are an extremely valuable national resource and they should be utilized in a manner that will protect as well as enhance, that national resource.

To summarize, I have briefly described our programs and goals in training and regulatory functions. I am fully aware that our regulatory functions are almost nonexistent and that participation in our training programs is completely voluntary. We are not reaching those laboratories whose directors object to any relationship with state agencies and label the program as government intervention in the private practice of medicine. Neither are we reaching those laboratories who fear an outside observation of their performance. However, these two groups are rapidly shrinking in numbers. The climate of professional attitudes toward licensure in Iowa is sufficiently negative at this time that it would be foolish to promote licensure legislation. Good things come to those who, with patience, wait. I am determined to wait.

LITERATURE CITED

1. Cheever, J. M. 1974. Travel and Leisure. American Express Company. Sept.
2. Center for Disease Control. 1970. Educational Opportunities for Laboratory Personnel. A National Directory of In-Service Continuing Educational Opportunities for Health Laboratory Personnel. Department of Health, Education, and Welfare, Atlanta.

SECTION II

Systems for
the Detection
and Identification
of Microorganisms

Introduction

George W. Campbell

A pathologist with whom I work is fond of saying, "When is microbiology going to enter the twentieth century?" He was, of course, referring to clinical microbiology. To paraphrase a popular commercial, "We've come a long way baby."

As this symposium demonstrates, we have moved away from reliance on morphology, staining, and fermentation of carbohydrates into an era where techniques such as enzymatic chemistry, fluorescence microscopy, immunoflurescence, radioisotopes, bioluminescence, gas-liquid chromatography, immunoelectrophoresis, radioimmunoassay (RIA), computers, and automation have penetrated into clinical microbiological laboratories.

We can now receive a specimen in the laboratory and detect the presence of organisms radiometrically within a few hours. Fluorescent microscopy enables us to detect mycobacteria in sputa and tissue much more rapidly, and probably more accurately than with acid-fast staining. Immunofluorescence enables us to detect pathogenic organisms in sputa, urethral discharges, etc., well before organisms are detectable by cultural techniques. Gas-liquid chromatography has provided us with the opportunity to identify organisms, particularly anaerobes, more rapidly and accurately than before. Immunoelectrophoresis is widely used in the detection of Australia antigen. RIA is being used for the assay of serum levels of antibiotics and shows promise in some other areas as well.

All of the foregoing are means of gathering information. In order to digest and evaluate the information, we have introduced the computer, which can handle enormous volumes of material in a very short time. If skilled programming is used, the resultant information can be used to great advantage in epidemiology, nosocomial infections, and also in speeding the identification procedures.

We have also been provided with something else in the way of modern innovations—the "kit." Almost all of these devices has, in one way or another, been packaged by the manufacturer into a form described as "easy to use." In a few cases, the manufacturer's claim seems to be true. If the manufacturer is competent and conscientious, the resultant kits provide a degree of uniformity and quality control which is difficult for any individual user to duplicate efficiently. On the other hand, if the manufacturer is careless or unscrupulous, numerous errors and misinterpretations can result from complete reliance on the kits or prepackaged systems.

Each new method, regardless of its form, should be compared to the best available methodology in current use. The user should determine a series of answers to questions such as:

1. Is this method accurate?
2. Is this method as reproducible?
3. Is this method as rapid?
4. Is this method as expensive?
5. Is this method likely to become quickly obsolescent?

The answers to these and other questions must be examined carefully before exchanging one methodology for another.

What may not be so obvious in the examination of new methods and equipment is that there has been a concurrent change in the people involved in clinical microbiology. The clinical microbiologist of 1974 is quite different from his predecessor of some years past.

The philosophy of the nature of disease has modified and evolved to the point where many microbiologists now view the process as change in the dynamic balance of microflora associated with humans. The analogy to ecological study is obvious. This dynamic balance can, of course, be altered by innumerable intrinsic and extrinsic factors. These factors are being vigorously explored in many aspects. The clinician of today relies on interpretation of microbiological information to a much greater degree than did his predecessor. Therefore, the microbiologist should become actively involved with clinicians and their problems and be an active consultant. This requires intelligence, empathy, and sometimes great restraint.

Although clinical microbiology has come a long way in a relatively short period, there still is need for further progress. Our speed of detection of some microorganisms is still terribly slow; in some cases, indeed, the best we can expect is a retrospective diagnosis. Even with numerous identification techniques and the services of computers, there still remain genera of uncertain affiliation. Perhaps an entirely different method of classification is needed.

The area of antimicrobial susceptibility testing is still in the horse and buggy days, even though somewhat heroic efforts have been made to reach a degree of standardization. Faced with equally or more difficult problems, our forebears found solutions. It is axiomatic in our society that the standard method of today becomes the obsolete method tomorrow. For some people, this has produced a phenomenon called "future shock," or the inability to adapt to rapid change. To these persons the changes we will discuss here pose something of a threat to the security of their status quo. To those with an eye to the future and an appreciation of the need for progress, this may really be the beginning of a new revolution in clinical microbiology. Whatever your viewpoint, there is no question that clinical microbiologists have the opportunity to do a better job than has been done in the past. We sometimes tend to fall victim to a very ancient disease at times like these and become so addicted to the instrument that we forget that the instrument is simply a tool to better understanding.

CHAPTER 4

Rapid Systems for the Detection of Bacteria and/or Their Products from Clinical Specimens

William J. Martin

In recent years there has been a tremendous surge of interest in the development of new systems along with a bewildering array of devices and approaches toward rapid detection and "easier" identification of microorganisms. Some of these systems such as gas-liquid chromatography (GLC) and the fluorescent antibody (FA) test have withstood the "test of time" and have become an integral part of the laboratory procedure, particularly in the larger laboratory. Others, through evaluation and use, are in various stages of evolution and, because of this, are going through a certain amount of revision. No doubt other methodologies are in the process of development, and there is every reason to believe that we, as microbiologists, can expect a diverse array of technology or hardware designed primarily to make life a little easier for us in the laboratory without sacrificing accuracy or economy in the process.

Rapid diagnosis of life-threatening infections due to the presence of bacteria or one or more of their products from clinical specimens is of the utmost importance. Obviously, such diagnosis depends primarily on the means employed for detection, as well as the subsequent identification procedures that may be used which enables the microbiologist to characterize the organism. Several of the more promising approaches currently being used or under investigation for consideration in the clinical microbiology laboratory are described here.

MICROBIAL-ANTIGEN DETECTION

An area that is receiving much attention lately in several laboratories as a means for rapid diagnosis of infections is microbial-antigen detection. By employing either gel-diffusion or counterimmunoelectrophoresis, diagnosis can be very rapid. Indeed, Greenwood, Whittle, and Dominic-Rajkovic (1), using counterimmunoelectrophoresis, detected meningococcal antigen within 45 min in the cerebrospinal fluid of 41 patients of whom only 17 had specimens which contained visible bacteria; all 41 proved to be culturally positive.

Microbial-antigen detection procedures appear to offer certain other advantages over traditional culture techniques. Besides speed, it seems to provide a good indication of pathogenicity, such as infections associated with the respiratory tract. Verhoef and Jones (2) found a relationship between the presence of pneumococcal antigens in sputum, the number of viable *Streptococcus pneumoniae,* and the severity of the disease. However, it should be noted that, in the experience of Spencer and Savage (3), patients with postoperative productive coughs were as likely to have antigen in their sputum as those with pneumonia. Although more investigations are needed in this area, it would seem to indicate that the presence of microbial antigen suggests a heavy bacterial infection and, therefore, implies infection rather than surface colonization.

If the implicated organism cannot be isolated from an infectious process, microbial-antigen detection has been employed and through implication the presence of bacteria has been shown. Inadequate inoculum, prior therapy, overgrowth by other microorganisms, and lack of suitable culture media all can be responsible for a lack of in vitro growth. In vivo, it has been shown that the diagnosis of primary pneumonia can be confused by overgrowth or by prior antimicrobial therapy. However, Tugwell and Greenwood (4) recently reported their observations that pneumococcal antigen can be detected in sputum even after treatment.

Other methods under evaluation for microbial-antigen detection include osmophoresis, reverse passive agglutination of antibody-coated latex particles, inhibition of passive hemagglutination, and radioimmunoassay. The latter technique can detect picogrammes of antigens. Whatever the methodology, they all depend on high-titered, specific antiserums. Indeed, many of the commercial antiserums were made for purposes other than these and, therefore, are inadequate. Bartram et al. (5) evaluated the sensitivity and specificity of osmophresis by testing serums from patients with pneumococcal pneumonia and bronchitis or various bacteremias, as well as extracts obtained from various bacterial cultures. These investigators used both a number of commercial and their own antiserums and found pneumococcal antigen in 54% of the patients with pneumonia. None was detected in their controls. Many of their bacteremic patients were noted to have an antigen in their blood. Moreover, an antigen was also present in the blood of 11 of their 12 patients with severe *Pseudomonas* infections. Tests with their laboratory cultures showed various cross-reactions with some of their pneumococcal antiserums reacting with four other species. These authors concluded that the difference between the in vitro and in vivo results was due to higher antigen concentrations in vitro. They further concluded that although their in vivo results were specific, occasional cross-reactions can occur. No doubt, results such as these are encouraging, but more experimental evidence will be needed to determine whether this technique can be relied upon as a laboratory test for routine use.

IMPEDANCE MEASUREMENTS

That growth of a few microorganisms can be detected by the change of electrical impedance in the culture has been advocated by Cady and his associates (6, 7). According to these investigators, impedance measurements provide a new method for measuring microorganism metabolism and growth. The device for recording these impedance changes, called a Bactometer, is capable of measuring the rate of bacterial metabolism and growth in less than 1 hour.

Growth curves appear to be produced rapidly by this method and vary with different species of bacteria. For example, Lawless, Dufour, and Cady (7) reported that impedance measurements in various sugar substrates can be used as part of an automated test for *Neisseria gonorrhoeae*. It was of interest that the addition of specific antigonococcal antiserum appeared to inhibit impedance response of their strains of *N. gonorrhoeae* in the 0 to 20-hour time span, with a resumption in normal response thereafter.

The early detection of bacterial growth by measurements of electrical impedance in blood cultures has been reported recently by Hadley and co-workers (8). They found the Bactometer to be a sensitive instrument that can detect evidence of bacterial activity when approximately 10^6 to 10^7 bacteria/ml are present. The Bactometer also can monitor up to 64 test cultures rapidly with little or no technologist attention. Moreover, the point recorder provides a continuous record of each culture with growth curves appearing as indicated by decreased impedance. Although host cells present in their blood cultures produced some impedance change by present reference methods, the authors felt that this did not inhibit early detection of bacteria at 5 to 10 hours in a blood culture.

Other uses for the Bactometer which appear to hold promise include the effect of antibiotics upon bacterial growth and the detection of mycoplasma, urinary tract pathogens in urine, and beer spoiling organisms in unpasteurized beer (6). Indeed, automated impedance measurements appear to provide a versatile tool, not only for rapid detection and characterization of microorganisms, but for use in immunology and biochemistry as well. Several evaluations of this method for detecting microorganisms are either planned or in progress (Cady, personal communication) and it remains to be seen whether this approach will offer any real advantage(s) over other techniques presently in use or under development.

MICROCALORIMETRY

It has been shown by Forrest (9) and other workers that data can be obtained by microcalorimetry of growing cultures as a result of bacterial metabolism. More recently, Boling, Blanchard, and Russell (10) applied microcalorimetry as a means of differentiating one microbial species from another, thereby obtaining characteristic profiles for different members of the family Enterobacteriaceae by observing the heat produced during their growth in liquid media.

Using a sample volume of 4 ml and observing growth of the organisms in brain-heart infusion (BHI) over periods of 8 to 14 hours, Boling, Blanchard, and Russell (10) obtained curves of heat production against time. Although Forrest (9) found that heat production ceased abruptly following the exhaustion of available glucose by *Streptococcus faecalis,* these investigators were able to show the same phenomenon for that organism in BHI. They further noted that curves for a given organism were virtually superimposable in repetitive experiments. Furthermore, these curves could differentiate all of their Enterobacteriaceae which included 17 species from 10 genera. For example, *Enterobacter aerogenes* and *Klebsiella* were clearly different in respect to their heat production, whereas some of their strains of *E. cloacae* could be separated from each other, although some possessed characteristics which permitted species identification.

Bacterial identification by microcalorimetry indicated to these workers that this approach provides a means for rapid and specific characterization of members of the family Enterobacteriaceae. They further acknowledged that organisms which do not grow well in broth cultures because of special metabolic needs did present problems that needed to be solved. However, for the majority of bacteria that should be identified in the routine laboratory, this method represented a powerful tool.

GAS-LIQUID CHROMATOGRAPHY

No doubt one of the more important advances that is currently taking place in the laboratory is the use of GLC as an aid in the identification of bacteria. Largely due to the efforts of several investigative groups in this country, gas chromatographic analysis of metabolic products has been shown to contribute significantly in the identification of bacteria. Indeed, analyses by GLC are not only simple and reliable for routine use but also are practical and desirable.

The use of direct GLC analysis of clinical specimens as a means for rapid detection of *Bacteroides fragilis* has been recently reported by Gorbach and his co-workers (11). Knowing that anaerobic bacteria produce specific short chain fatty acids from carbohydrate metabolism, these workers directly analyzed 65 clinical specimens, such as pus and serous fluid, by simple acidification or methylation and GLC. The specimens also were cultured by aerobic and anaerobic methods. They found good correlation with isobutyric (ib), butyric (b), and succinic (s) acids. Of 11 pus specimens that eventually grew *B. fragilis,* all had ib, b, and s acids by direct analysis. Only one specimen, a putrid empyema, had ib, b, and s acids but failed to grow a Gram negative anaerobe despite clinical and Gram stain impressions. These authors further reported that no s and only small amounts of ib and b acids were detected in 18 pus and infected serous fluids with coliforms, *Pseudomonas,* staphylococci, facultative, and anaerobic streptococci, and *Clostridium.* No acids were detected in 35 sterile specimens of pleural, peritoneal, and joint fluid. They concluded that the only false positive was probably a failure of culture techniques in a putrid empyema specimen. They further concluded that the combination of s, ib, and b acids is a useful fingerprint to detect the presence of *B. fragilis* in clinical specimens. These fatty acids can be directly analyzed by GLC, and a presumptive diagnosis can be made within 1 hr of collection.

In another recent study from this laboratory, Mayhew et al. (12) reported on direct GLC analysis of clinical specimens for rapid detection of strepto-cocci. By measuring the end product, lactic acid (LA), 63 clinical specimens were Gram stained and cultured aerobically, under CO_2, and anaerobically. LA was determined in the specimen by GLC analysis following acidification, methylation, and chloroform extraction. Their results were studied in a "blind" fashion and 20 specimens showed both Gram positive cocci on smear and greater than 0.2 meq/100 ml LA. Streptococci were cultured in 18, with the remaining 2 specimens being obtained from patients receiving antibiotics which may have prevented recovery of this organism. Forty-one of 43 specimens which failed to meet both criteria had negative cultures for streptococci; these organisms in the remaining 2 were judged by these investigators as not clinically significant and may have been contaminants. Neither LA determination nor Gram stain alone proved satisfactory for accurate prediction of eventual culture. It was indicated from these findings that LA analysis in combination with Gram stain may prove useful for rapid detection of streptococci in clinical material.

Another very recent study on the promising application of GLC as a means for the rapid detection of bacteria from clinical specimens was re-ported by Brooks et al. (13). Employing GLC as a potential means of diagnosing arthritis, these workers were able to differentiate between staphylococcal, streptococcal, gonococcal, and traumatic arthritis. Both acidic and basic extracts of synovial fluids from patients with well-documented cases of arthritis were studied using a gas chromatograph equipped with an electron-capture detector. They obtained profiles which were sufficiently dissimilar to permit differentiation between synovitis caused by trauma and that caused by staphylococcal, streptococcal, and gonococcal infections. Their in vitro studies included incubation of the bacterial isolates in control synovial fluids and comparison of resulting profiles obtained from the in vivo studies. Gas chromatography data from both the in vitro studies and studies of samples taken after effective antibiotic therapy indicated that many of the volatile components detected from diseased synovial fluids were metabolites of the pathogenic agent or metabolites of the host that had been modified by the presence of the parasite. They concluded from their data that GLC might be used to help determine the etiology of various types of arthritis.

Analyzing sugars in normal and infected cerebrospinal fluid by GLC has been recently shown by Amundson, Braude, and Davis (14) to be a highly reproducible procedure. Analysis of trimethylsilyl derivatives of 14 normal human cerebrospinal fluid samples were found to contain α- and β-glucose as well as isomers of two unidentified sugars. They noted chromatographic changes in three cases of meningeal inflammation—two cryptococcosis and one thalamic astrocytoma—which were limited to decreased concentrations of all sugars. Moreover, in one case of early meningitis, the concentrations of the unknown sugars decreased before glucose. Since a reproducible chromatogram of the trimethylsilyl derivatives of normal cerebrospinal fluid had been established by these investigators, it was felt that more samples of abnormal cerebrospinal fluid should be prepared by these methods and examined by GLC.

From these, as well as other, observations, the use of GLC has, in my opinion, tremendous potential in the diagnostic laboratory for rapid diagnosis of infections, particularly those which may be caused by organisms which are difficult to isolate and identify or are not rapidly grown.

LIMULUS TEST

Gelation of a lysate of the blood cells (amebocytes) of the horseshoe crab, limulus, with low concentrations of endotoxins, lipopolysaccharides that form a portion of the cell walls of Gram negative bacteria, has led to the development of an assay capable of detecting less than nanogram concentrations of endotoxin in human blood (15). Because of its sensitivity, as well as its apparent specificity, a simple in vitro test has been developed by Levin and associates (15, 16). Employing this test, these investigators have suggested that such a rapid assay for endotoxin can be of diagnostic value in infections with Gram negative bacilli. They further felt that a correlation existed between a positive assay and the occurrence of shock and death in such infections.

Several additional reports from other laboratories have confirmed the usefulness of the limulus test in detecting endotoxin in small amounts not only from blood but also from other clinical specimens. For example, Nachum, Lipsey, and Siegel (17) evaluated the limulus test as a means for the rapid diagnosis of Gram negative bacterial meningitis. They found the assay to be a rapid, sensitive test for the diagnosis of untreated Gram negative bacterial meningitis and found that it may be useful for the detection of persistent bacterial growth or residual endotoxin in the presence of other spinal fluid abnormalities. Although the kinds of Gram negative bacteria encountered in their study was rather limited, results of limulus tests of urine as well as plasma samples from patients with infections due to a wide range of Gram negative organisms suggests similar reliability (15, 18).

In a recent report, Stumacher, Kovenat, and McCabe (19) reported that the limulus test detected endotoxin or endotoxin-like material in the blood of almost 50% of their patients with bacteremia due to Gram negative bacilli, and in 26% of patients with nonbacteremic infections with Gram negative organisms. These workers further observed that the blood of 36% of their patients with Gram positive bacteremia also produced positive limulus tests. Since no concomitant infection with Gram negative bacteria was observed in these latter patients, the diagnostic value of this assay was seriously questioned by these authors. Moreover, they found no correlation between positive assays and the number of circulating Gram negative bacilli or the occurrence of shock and death. Levin et al. (15), on the other hand, reported negative limulus tests in all 25 of their patients with a variety of bacteremias due to Gram positive organisms, including staphylococci, streptococci, and pneumococci. Obviously, additional study will have to be forthcoming in order to try to resolve this important discrepancy.

"False-negative" limulus tests also have been the subject of numerous reports, particularly on plasma obtained from patients with documented Gram negative bacteremia (15, 16, 20, 21). Indeed, detection of endotoxin in plasma has presented a number of practical and theoretical difficulties, i.e., chloroform extraction of the plasma inhibitor, effects on the dilution of the relatively larger plasma volume, etc. At this point, it might be appropriate to quote from a recent editorial on the subject by Dr. Levin which appeared in the *New England Journal of Medicine* (20): "Current problems with the limulus test consist of technique and standardization, and better methods are needed to resolve the efficacy and specificity of this test, and to determine whether the results obtained correlate with changes that have been attributed to endotoxemia. Final evaluation of the specificity of the limulus test awaits the development of another, equally sensitive assay and one that does not depend on a biologic activity of endotoxin."

MINI-CULTURE METHODS FOR DETECTION OF BACTERIURIA

No doubt one of the most widely accepted procedures in the diagnostic laboratory is the use of quantitative bacterial culture methods for differentiating true bacteriuria from contamination of the urine specimen with urethral flora during micturation. Although the calibrated loop and plate culture method is used by most laboratories, it does have some practical disadvantages. For example, prompt delivery of the specimen to the laboratory or, at least, refrigeration of the specimen until it is cultured is definitely required for proper quantitation. In addition, properly trained personnel in diagnostic bacteriology are needed. It is not unexpected, therefore, that several approaches to try to alleviate some of these disadvantages in detecting bacteriuria have been marketed in recent years.

One of the initial approaches was the availability of relatively cheap, efficient, and accurate dip-inoculum methods for urine cultures. Through the years, a number of dip-inoculum tests have been developed beginning with a simple glass slide coated on one end with selective agar (22) to those containing agar-filled wells and paddles and agar-coated pipettes (23, 24). In many instances, these methods compared quite favorably with the standard pour plate procedure and were reported under certain circumstances to be more accurate than the calibrated loop method (25, 26). Because the presently available dip-inoculum methods require not only refrigeration of test materials but also time for incubation, a need still existed for a rapid, cheap, and accurate test for detecting bacteriuria.

Such a test has recently come on the market which appears to combine both chemical and bacteriological methods. Employing a small plastic strip that is capable of indefinite storage, it is called the Dip-Incubate-Read (DIR) method and is marketed as Microstix (Ames Co., Elkhart, Indiana). It consists of a clear polystyrene strip with two dehydrated culture media areas along with a nitrite reagent area arranged in sequence at one end.

In a recent evaluation of this dip-inoculum method for detecting bacteriuria in hospitalized patients, Moffat, Britt, and Burke (27) directly compared results from both quantitative cultures and the Microstix test in 1,661 urine specimens. Discrepant interpretations were made by independent observers in 9.3% of the specimens with $>10^5$ colonies/ml. It was further observed that the media areas failed to support the growth of yeast and gave variable results with *Staphylococcus epidermidis* and non-group D streptococci. False-negative culture results commonly occurred if the patients were receiving antibiotics. These investigators found that the nitrite test remained occasionally positive for brief periods after the elimination of bacteriuria by antibiotics. Conditions and drugs (especially phenazopyridine) which discolor urine were noted to interfere with reading both the culture and nitrite tests. These workers concluded that the Microstix test strip, although not suitable for hospital use or for monitoring therapy, is probably as reliable as the calibrated loop method for office screening.

CONCLUSION

I have tried to provide a brief overview of what I consider to be the basic trends in design for the rapid detection of bacteria and/or their products from clinical specimens. Indeed, we as microbiologists are witnessing a mild revolution in the laboratory. Although perhaps not of the magnitude that has transformed the methodology in the clinical chemistry and hematology laboratories, similar technology is now finding application in the microbiology laboratory. Impressive as these detection systems appear to be for the most part, much more investigative work and many more evaluations will be needed to prove their worth in the laboratory on a day-to-day basis. Moreover, it remains to be seen how effective some of these systems, i.e., Bactomatic, microcalorimetry, etc., will be in the detection of individual bacterial species from a mixed population of microorganisms such as is frequently found in abdominal abscesses or wound infections. Furthermore, it should be stressed that, since most microbiology laboratories are simply not in the position to undertake programs to evaluate such systems, it becomes essential, for these laboratories to either assess the new systems themselves or await results of impartial and objective assessments by reference laboratories prior to using them.

LITERATURE CITED

1. Greenwood, B. M., H. C. Whittle, and O. Dominic-Rajkovic. 1971. Counter-current immunoelectrophoresis in the diagnosis of meningococcal infections. Lancet 11:519–521.
2. Verhoef, J., and D. M. Jones. 1974. Pneumococcal antigen in sputum (Letters to the Editor). Lancet 1:879.
3. Spencer, R. C., and M. A. Savage. 1974. Pneumococcal antigen in sputum (Letters to the Editor). Lancet 1:879.
4. Tugwell, R., and B. M. Greenwood. 1974. Bacteriological findings in pneumonia (Letters to the Editor). Lancet 1:95.
5. Bartram, C. E., J. G. Crowder, B. Beeler, and A. White. 1974. Diagnosis of bacterial diseases by detection of serum antigens by counterimmunoelectrophoresis, sensitivity, and specificity of detecting *Pseudomonas* and pneumococcal antigens. J. Lab. & Clin. Med. 83:591–598.
6. Cady, P., S. W. Dufour, and D. Thornton. 1974. An impedance approach

to automating bacteriology. Presented at the Association for the Advancement of Medical Instrumentation Annual Meeting, April, 1974.

7. Lawless, P., S. Dufour, and P. Cady. 1973. Impedance changes in media as a method of identifying microorganisms. Presented at the International Congress in Bacteriology, Tel Aviv, Israel, September 2—7, 1973.

8. Hadley, W. K., G. Seny K, R. Michaels, and J. Seman. 1974. Early detection of bacterial growth by measurements of electrical impedance in blood cultures. Abstr. of the Annual Meeting of the American Society for Microbiology, M281.

9. Forrest, W. W. 1972. Microcalorimetry. J. R. Norris, and D. W. Ribbons (ed.), Methods in Microbiology, 6B:285. Academic Press, New York.

10. Boling, E. A., G. C. Blanchard, and W. J. Russell. 1973. Bacterial identification by microcalorimetry. Nature 241:472—473.

11. Gorbach, S. L., J. W. Mayhew, J. G. Bartlett, H. Thadepalli, and A. B. Onderdonk. 1974. Rapid diagnosis of *Bacteroides fragilis* infections by direct gas liquid chromatography of clinical specimens. Abstr. Clin. Res. 22:442A.

12. Mayhew, J. W., A. Onderdonk, J. Bartlett, and S. L. Gorbach. 1974. Direct gas-liquid chromatographic (GLC) analysis of clinical material for rapid detection of streptococci. Abstract of the Annual Meeting of the American Society for Microbiology, M47.

13. Brooks, J. B., D. S. Kellogg, C. C. Alley, H. B. Short, H. H. Handsfield, and B. Huff. 1974. Gas chromatography as a potential means of diagnosing arthritis. I. Differentiation between staphylococcal, streptococcal, gonococcal, and traumatic arthritis. J. Infect. Dis. 129:660—668.

14. Amundson, S., A. I. Braude, and C. E. Davis. 1974. Rapid diagnosis of infection by gas-liquid chromatography: analysis of sugars in normal and infected cerebrospinal fluid. Appl. Microbiol. 28:298—302.

15. Levin, J., T. E. Poore, N. J. Young, S. Margolis, N. P. Zauber, A. S. Townes, and W. R. Bell. 1972. Gram-negative sepsis: Detection of endotoxemia with the limulus test: With studies of associated changes in blood coagulation, serum lipids, and complement. Ann. Int. Med. 76:1—7.

16. Levin, J., T. E. Poore, N. P. Zauber, and R. S. Oser. 1970. Detection of endotoxin in the blood of patients with sepsis due to gram-negative bacteria. New England J. Med. 283:1313—1316.

17. Nachum, R., A. Lipsey, and S. E. Siegel. 1973. Detection of gram-negative bacterial meningitis by limulus lysate test. New England J. Med. 289:931—934.

18. Jorgensen, J. H., H. F. Carvajal, B. E. Chipps, and R. F. Smith. 1973. Rapid detection of gram-negative bacteriuria by use of the *Limulus* endotoxin assay. Appl. Microbiol. 26:38—42.

19. Stumacher, R. J., M. J. Kovenat, and W. R. McCabe. 1973. Limitations of the usefulness of the limulus assay for endotoxin. New England J. Med. 288:1261—1264.

20. Levin, J. 1973. Endotoxin and endotoxemia. New England J. Med. 288:1297—1298.

21. Martinez-G, L. A., R. Quintiliani, and R. C. Tilton. 1973. Clinical experience on the detection of endotoxemia with the limulus test. J. Infect. Dis. 127:102—105.

22. Cohen, S. N., and E. H. Kass. 1967. A simple method for quantitative urine culture. New England J. Med. 277:176—180.

23. Craig, W. A., and C. M. Kunin. 1972. Quantitative urine culture method using a plastic "paddle" containing dual media. Appl. Microbiol. 23:919–922.

24. Kunin, C. M., and J. A. Bergeron. 1972. A simple quantitative urine culture method using an internally coated plastic pipette. Am. J. Clin. Path. 58:371–375.

25. McAllister, T. A. 1973. The day of the dipslide. Nephron 11:123–133.

26. McAllister, T. A., G. C. Arneil, W. Barr, and P. Kay. 1973. Assessment of plane dipslide quantitation of bacteriuria. Nephron 11:111–122.

27. Moffat, C. M., M. R. Britt, and J. P. Burke. 1974. Evaluation of miniature test for bacteriuria using dehydrated media and nitrite pads. Appl. Microbiol. 28:95–99.

CHAPTER 5

Biochemical "Rapid Identification" of Enterobacteriaceae

Henry D. Isenberg

Clinical microbiologists have grown accustomed to the term rapid identification and understand it to refer to the various commercially manufactured kits or system approaches for the recognition of the various medically significant members of the family *Enterobacteriaceae*. This designation reflects, of course, the shortcomings of words to describe a given set of conditions. One need not belabor the point. It is obvious, especially to the semantic and scientific purist, that these approaches are not rapid in the sense that the time required to obtain results has been reduced. Identification is accomplished in the diagnostic, non-adonsonian sense rather than on the level of the classic taxonomists. Parenthetically, anyone who has seen the latest contribution to the obfuscation of bacterial nomenclature in the form of the most recent edition of Bergey's Manual (1) will be delighted with the reasonable and intelligent fashion with which clinical microbiologists treat this particular family of procaryotes. It is only fitting and proper that, at the onset of this discussion, we all acknowledge our limitless indebtedness to the genius of William Ewing for having brought order and clarity to the chaotic confusion which persisted in this family since the very beginning of diagnostic bacteriology.

It may not be considered within the scope of this meeting, but I do feel compelled to spend the time to remind all of us that even modern taxonomy fails almost completely at the protistal and especially at the procaryotic level

41

of life. We must recognize what I have referred to in the past as a biological uncertainty principle, a concession on the part of microbiologists that we really do not know exactly what a bacterium is. Those of you who are convinced that I exaggerate our collective state of ignorance, I would implore to remember the statement of Stanier and Van Niel (2), who said in 1962, "Any good biologist finds it intellectually distressing to devote his life to the study of a group that cannot be readily and satisfactorily defined in biological terms; the abiding intellectual scandal of bacteriology has been the absence of a clear concept of the bacterium." Nothing has happened in the interim to modify this admission by two of the great microbiologists. We do not deal with the individual bacterium at any time; to be sure, our study of the vast populations that we treat as if they were individuals is based on the assumption that they are the progeny of the single individual bacterium which finds itself in the most unnatural fashion isolated on an artificial substrate inside a petri dish. Without meaning to, we then deny all levels of variation, selection, classical genetics and molecular biology and proceed with a million as if they were but that single bacterium we cannot define. Then we expose the object of our transient interest to a variety of substrates to assess its physiological attributes and attempt to fit these reactions into a pattern we have all agreed denotes "species." Should we want to be more convincing, we corroborate our identification with a more or less complex mixture of animal immuno-globulins, occasionally even adorned with a fluorescent dye, and, thus, the concerned clinician with irrefutable proof of the correctness of our results.

It is no consolation that we seem to be right most of the time. No one can prove us wrong since no one knows any better way to achieve tagging the large population with another more accurate designation. We should keep in mind the first figure in the original Edwards and Ewing volume (3) on the family *Enterobacteriaceae*. It depicted a large circle, the family. This large circle encompassed the facultative anaerobic, Gram-negative, peritrichously flagellated rods carrying antigens in a mosaic pattern and capable of produc-ing catalase and nitrate reductase, but not oxidase. Within this circle there were numerous small ones. These circles designated the genera within the family, collected by additionally shared biochemical activities. The authors pointed out that there was no abrupt division between the population densities sharing properties. Instead, while many bacteria populate the dense areas and are identified with ease, many others display activities which place them in intermediate positions. Since phylogenetic analysis of any bacterium is prevented not only by bacterial insistence on a haploid state but also by its totally indiscriminate mating patterns which transcend alleged genus, tribe, and family boundaries, we ought to begin to regard all prokaryotes as a continuum of living forms capable of all the various biochemical and physio-logical activities which are required for supporting the metastable state we call life. To offset this depressing and discouraging observation, we do know that we can use a series of biochemical activities and physiological responses to sequester and recognize bacteria from vast mixtures of microorganisms. Practical diagnostic taxonomy is an important tool in delineating the normal and pathological role of the microbiota in the intimate biosphere of the human host. We may not know or understand all of the theoretical implications or foundations of our endeavors. We know they work—and most often for the benefit of patients and the community.

Differentiation of bacteria one from the other on the basis of biochemical activities is probably one of the oldest approaches to the study of these forms. Since the microscopic dimensions and paucity of morphological alternatives hampered the scientific analysis of bacteria in the last century, their great biochemical productivity was recognized as a most significant attribute for their classification. While there was considerable preoccupation with the causal relationships between specific microorganisms and disease, the early assessment of biochemical differences reflects the great concern with the sanitary supply of water, waste disposal, and contamination of foods. Thus, the family *Enterobacteriaceae* has been, and still is, at the very heart of the evaluation of biochemical taxonomy of microorganisms. The nature of these organisms generated the underlying concept of modern clinical microbiology—namely, the demonstration of clear-cut differences between those populations we call species in the most reproducible, accurate, and expeditious manner. What modern microbiologists have forgotten is the appreciation by their professional predecessors of the natural distribution of the family *Enterobacteriaceae*. Ninety years ago it was known that some of the members of what we now call the family Enterobacteriaceae were residents of man and animals, while others inhabited soil, plants, and muds. This distinction led to four major categories of biochemical characterizations. These are (a) fermentation, (b) end product recognition, (c) use of indicators and buffers, and (d) inducible enzymes. These divisions parallel the physiological exploration of intermediary metabolism of carbohydrates and energy in general and they serve as another example of the pioneering role of microbiologists in the elucidation of biological processes. The enzyme tests such as those for the various decarboxylases are more recent and represent a growing appreciation among scientists of cellular control mechanisms.

The so-called "system approaches" or "rapid systems" are no departure from the classical tests which accumulated during the last 90 years in attempts to identify and speciate members of the family. These systems represent the judicious selection of substrates to ensure reproducible and slightly more rapid results in the identification process. Their major time-saving aspect is the reduction in preparatory labor, glassware, and media. To this one must add the comparative ease with which the literature accompanying the various systems' approaches guide the technical staff through the maze of taxonomy and reactions and allow even neophytes to arrive at comparatively accurate identifications. There are 4 major systems presently in use.

1. *The r/b system* represents a unique formulation of 14 biochemical parameters into a series of 4 tubes. There is no division between the various media contained in any 1 tube, requiring a careful formulation of the substrate combined into any 1 tube. The 4 tubes are all characterized by carrying a physical modification in the tube, i.e., a constriction which enables some additional physical separation of substrates which might diffuse into one another and confuse clear-cut results. This system's first tube contains in the slant the phenylalanine deaminase reactants and lactose fermentation reagents; in the upper bud, hydrogen sulfide production can be noted as well as glucose fermentation and gas production. The lower bud carries the reactants for lysine decarboxylase. This reaction is separated from the others by the constriction provided in this first tube. The second tube, smaller in dimension, serves for the testing of the indole in the upper part of the semisolid medium. The constricted portion holds the reaction for ornithine decarboxylase while motility can be assessed in the general appearance of both. The third tube, usually included in the initial screens for the identification of members of the family, carries citrate in the upper portion and rhamnose fermentation indicators in the lower portion of the tube. The fourth and final tube in the system, used whenever reactions in the first three indicate the need for additional tests, is divided into a section for detection of DNase production and raffinose fermentation in the slant. The upper bud carries sorbitol and the indicator denotes its fermentation while the constricted portion carries arabinose. The uses and application of the system to the identification of members of the family *Enterobacteriaceae* have been studied in several laboratories and its performance has been excellent. It has been estimated in a series of comparison studies to perform at the 95–98% level of efficiency in identifying the various members of the family encountered in clinical specimens. Results are read in a standardized fashion which leads to the elimination of a number of possibilities by virtue of the reactions and the arrangement for reading the responses. Recently a small, ingenious electronic device has been introduced called the Enteric Analyzer which enables the technical staff to ascertain the identity of various organisms at the 90% and 99% level. The instrument provides a series of additional tests in order to identify the rarely occurring abnormal biotype or those members of the family *Enterobacteriaceae* infrequently encountered in the intimate human biosphere.

2. *The improved enterotube* employs 10 significant biochemical substrates separated from one another into 8 compartments, all contained within a single tube. The tube is inoculated with a wire provided in the kit which will insure the distribution of organisms to each of the compartments by withdrawing this wire after it has been in contact with a single colony on any one of the selective or nonselective media usually employed in the clinical

laboratory. In this system, fermentation of glucose and gas production of glucose is assessed along with the determination of lysine decarboxylase, ornithine decarboxylase, the production of hydrogen sulfide and indole, lactose as well as dulcitol fermentation, phenylalanine deaminase, urease production, and citrate utilization. Schemes for the identification of organisms are provided. The matter of reporting can be performed in several ways. There is provision for rendering results in computer language or in a manner which generates a 4-digit number. The 4-digit identification number can be referred to a reference manual containing identifications of various members of the family gathered from a very broad information base. In the event that several different organisms might provide the same 10 initial tests and cannot be differentiated from one another on that basis, suggestions for additional biochemical examinations are provided. This reference system, known as Encise II, also has the novel feature of providing information on the likelihood that each organism may give the reactions which led to this final numeric result. The individual laboratory worker may then choose to perform the additional biochemical tests or to be satisfied with the differences in the likelihood and report the most likely organism. This system has been studied in great detail in several laboratories. It performs at the level of 95 to 98% efficiency in recognizing the organisms encountered in the clinical microbiology laboratory.

3. *The API (Analylab Products Inc.) system* provides the laboratory with 20 microtubes carrying the following substrates: ONPG, arginine dihydrolase, lysine decarboxylase, ornithine decarboxylase, citrate, substrate for hydrogen sulfide demonstration, urease, tyrosine deaminase, substrate for indole production, substrate for the demonstration of the elaboration of acetylmethylcarbinol, gelatin liquification substrate, and fermentation substrates for glucose, mannitol, inositol, sorbitol, rhamnose, sucrose, melibiose, amygdalin, and arabinose. These various tests are combined on a unique cardboard strip which is incubated in its own plastic tray. A bacterial suspension is made in sterile distilled water and the mixture is added to the test vessels. Sterile mineral oil is added to close off the tube opening, described as a cupule by the manufacturer, for the reactions involving the dihydrolases, decarboxylases, and urease production. Guides for the proper reading of the tests are provided and organisms may be identified with the help of a profile register provided by the manufacturer after a numerical value is established with the use of an API coder. This system is backed by a very wide base of information available through a computer hook-up to all users who choose to avail themselves of this service. The printout by the computer informs the user of what additional tests may be required and what the likelihood is that these reactions indicate a specific species or biotype of the various members of the family *Enterobacteriaceae*. The performance of this system is at the level of 95 to 98% in the identification of these organisms.

Several other similar systems have been introduced. Some have been scrutinized very carefully by several laboratories and found not to perform at the level of the three mentioned commercial products. Several others are being tested and undoubtedly a large number of variations on the same theme will appear in the near future.

4. *The Minitek system* has not as yet been evaluated to the extent of the three systems described above. The system is novel in that it allows the laboratory to choose the various substrates to be tested. This system is provided with a dispenser which holds substrates in a fashion similar to that for the dispensing of antibiotics. A special plate containing 10 wells is provided. An inoculum is prepared in a special broth which is dispensed with an automatic pipette provided with disposable tips. Adding the plate to the dispenser releases the substrates desired. The plate cover is replaced and several plates are incubated in a special holder. Reactions may then be read at the appropriate time. While the system has not been fully evaluated, it promises to provide the type of flexibility so important to most clinical microbiologists.

While these systems may differ in their formulations, the number and complexity of the reactions involved, and the physical means of providing the substrate, they share certain advantages. Perhaps the most significant advantage is the opportunity to provide the clinical microbiology laboratory with standardized material. All can utilize the same reaction and the same reagents and, hopefully, follow the same procedure in order to perform each of these tests. This is a most desirable departure from the use of the so-called "conventional" systems since each laboratory usually introduces its own modifications.

Another advantage is that the systems employ the "quick decision" reactions for the identification of the members of the family. None of the systems incorporates reagents which require 7, 10, or even 21 days to elicit a reaction for the identification of the organisms. Thus, the systems approach provides a shortening of the time period for the identification of significant organisms. While the 24-hr reaction does not entitle any system to call itself rapid, quite obviously the thrust of the effort is to approach a shorter time period for the identification. Another advantage, inherent in commercially available systems approaches to the identification of medically significant microorganisms, is that many laboratories heretofore unable to provide this type of service to their clinicians will now be in a position to identify members of the family with alacrity. I am as aware as is this audience of the challenges recently stated about the need for this capability. There are those who would hold on to the principles of infectious disease enunciated in the latter part of the last century. There seems to be no doubt that the most pertinent information required by a physician to make a diagnosis and treat the patient does not necessarily involve species identity. There can be, however, no doubt also that, in our present society and our present medical facilities, with the nosocomial disease complications rising in frequency and potentially extending into the community, the identity of a microorganism means more than academic interest or the self-aggrandizement of clinical laboratory scientists. I do hope that the laboratory fraternity in medical institutions will resist strongly a neglectful analysis of any specimen. The responsibilities each of us carries not only toward the individual patient but also toward the hospital community at large, coupled with a rapid and easy identification of the microorganism to the species level, make it mandatory that these recent suggestions in the name of preserving funds and not providing too much information to the clinician be treated with the disdain they deserve.

The commercial systems provide a great assurance of reproducibility within each laboratory and from laboratory to laboratory utilizing the same reagent. This is perhaps an additional view of the observations made earlier that the commercial system enables the clinical microbiology laboratory to proceed in a more standardized fashion in the identification of this family.

While one would not hope that a prescription for one or another system would be forthcoming from a federal level, as happened with the testing for antibiotic susceptibility, nevertheless the advantage for standardized performance of examinations is very obvious and can be derived with great ease by the use of any one of the systems mentioned. These systems assure a quality of reagent which is especially significant to those laboratories which do not perform species identification with a frequency found in some select institutions. These approaches also set the stage for the expansion of this type of approach to other microbial groups of medical significance. Another significant role that these systems provide to the understanding of the family *Enterobacteriaceae* is that the data base on which identification is founded can be broadened considerably. I do not mean to detract in any way or manner from the contributions of Ewing in providing us with the percentage tables on the reactions of the various members of the family Enterobacteriaceae. However, we must acknowledge that the organisms on which these reactions are based were obtained from clinical specimens and, therefore, quite probably from those bacteria engaged in complicating disease processes. At this juncture we do not understand the selective influences of the environment in a diseased tissue which would encourage one particular species or several species of the family to proliferate in an abnormal body site. I want to point out merely that no one, including the commercial companies which provide these systems for speciation, has studied the reaction of "wild type" organisms found in various geographically separated areas in normal individuals and in normal locations. We are unaware of the reactions of *Escherichia coli,* for example, isolated from innumerable stools of perfectly normal individuals. No one has bothered or seen reason to bother with ascertaining the biochemical and physiological activities of such organisms. Our encounters with representatives of the genus *Enterobacter* have taken place within the medical setting; no one has looked recently at the variation in their activities when the organisms originated from their more normal and natural habitat in soil and on plants. This pertains to a large variety of other representatives which we identify on a percentage basis at this time. My opinion is that the number of abnormally reacting representatives will not decrease in the medical setting, but that a more realistic assessment of the frequency with which they occur in nature will result. This in itself might be significant in the clinical sense, for the biochemically anomalously reacting organism may, therefore, represent a selective process exerted by the host. The biochemical marker may carry much greater clinical significance than we assume at this time.

The problem of the rare biotype should be clarified. Perhaps these systems will allow the separation of the rarely occurring microorganisms. We may then also be able to prove that this variation has no real significance and that some of the labor expanded in pursuing the identification of such biotypes may be abandoned with impunity. It is also necessary to mention that the proper technical performance and proper controls must be conducted when commercial systems are employed. Unfortunately, none of the manufacturers has stressed that certain control organisms ought to be employed with each of the systems. A select few bacteria will certainly enable us to elicit positive and negative reactions for each of the parameters included in each system. It would seem desirable that every tenth or fifteenth set should be exposed to such control organisms.

There is a final statement I feel compelled to make. It concerns the transient nature of the systems approaches to the identification of microorganisms in a clinical laboratory. After many years of stagnation clinical microbiology technology is moving toward realizing its responsibility in providing accurate and rapid service to the clinician who requires this information for the diagnosis and the treatment of his patient. The goal we ought to set for ourselves is to accomplish this task within the usual working day of the laboratory. I mean that we should be able to identify and provide antibiograms to the clinician in the same fashion that the chemistry and hematology laboratories function for the benefit of the patient. It is in this sense that I feel the approach through the rapid biochemical systems is one that fills a stopgap and must be supplanted through the concerted efforts of all who work in the clinical laboratory. I feel strongly that the answer to this problem is not found in the computer and in the identification of rare types of organisms. I am also certain that mere mechanizations of technical tasks or even automation alone will not solve the problem. What is needed to identify members of this and all other microbial families are more sensitive devices for the detection of microbial end products, in other words, to bring 20th century technology to the problem of diagnostic clinical microbiology. We should also not ignore the advances of molecular biology and endeavor to bring some of the insights gained by this offspring of microbiology to bear on the problems confronting us in the infectious disease field. Our recognition of the unnatural fashion in which we have handled microorganisms to date is also most important. The pure culture concept must be supplanted if we wish to appreciate fully the polymicrobic infectious disease potential and the role it plays in many infectious disease manifestations. Finally we ought to begin to look at the body fluids of the patient himself and attempt to correlate alterations in these specimens with the presence of microorganisms. The recent advances in the application of gas liquid chromatography not only to the identification and speciation of anaerobic bacteria but also to body fluids and to culture supernatants indicate that the 24-hr time period could indeed be reduced to a 2- or 3-hr period. If this type of procedure could then be automated, we would begin to approach our noble goal, namely, to be of help in the more rapid diagnosis and treatment of infectious disease.

LITERATURE CITED

1. Buchanan, R. E., and N. E. Gibbons. 1974. Bergey's Manual of Determinative Bacteriology. Ed. 8. The Williams & Wilkins Co., Baltimore.
2. Stanier, R. Y., and C. B. van Niel. 1962. The concept of a bacterium. Arch. f. Mibrobiol. 42: 17—35.
3. Edwards, P. R., and W. H. Ewing. 1958. Identification of Enterobacteriaceae. Burgess Publishing Co., Minneapolis.

CHAPTER 6

Immunofluorescence Tests for Bacteria

William B. Cherry

Although immunofluorescence (IF) techniques have been available as diagnostic tools for 20 years, their acceptance as routine test procedures in the clinical or public health laboratory has been slow and disappointing. Close examination of the reasons for this indicates a complex interplay of scientific and economic factors. To be widely accepted, a new test procedure must be: (a) scientifically acceptable, (b) economically sound, and (c) productive of information, not otherwise obtainable, which is important to health care.

If one examines proposed IF tests with these requirements in mind, it is apparent that some have not been accepted for one or more of the reasons listed above. One example of a scientifically unacceptable IF test is staining nasopharyngeal smears with a conjugate for *Corynebacterium diphtheriae* for detection of the diphtheria bacillus. This application was unacceptable for two reasons: (a) the inability to produce an IF reagent which would, with reasonable accuracy, differentiate the diphtheria bacillus from other throat flora; and (b) the inability to differentiate toxigenic from nontoxigenic strains. Another IF test which has failed to measure up to its earlier promise is that for the diagnosis of gonorrhea. In this case the reagent used lacked the necessary specificity.

Determinations of economic feasibility have been affected by: (a) cost of IF equipment, (b) frequency of requests for performance of a particular IF test, (c) adequacy of personnel training, (d) availability of commercial IF

51

reagents of satisfactory quality, and (e) problems of laboratory operation related to work flow. The use of IF tests to detect *Mycobacterium tuberculosis* or to differentiate other mycobacteria has been severely limited by the unavailability of commercial reagents. Use of IF tests to aid in the diagnosis of plague, anthrax, tularemia, and melioidosis has been adversely affected by frequency of requests for performance of a particular IF test, adequacy of personnel training, and availability of commercial IF reagents of satisfactory quality.

The potential use of IF tests for the rapid, sensitive, and serologically specific diagnosis of meningitis due to meningococci, pneumococci, *Hemophilus influenzae,* and *Listeria* has not been realized because competent individuals can detect these organisms within the required time frame by using the simple Gram-stain procedure and by culture. IF tests will provide presumptive identification of these organisms with great reliability and sensitivity and with a rapidity comparable to that of the Gram stain. However, these advantages, which ultimately benefit the patient, have not been of sufficient primacy to insure widespread adoption of the IF tests. Undoubtedly, the complexity of the reagents and problems concerned with their availability and quality have influenced acceptance of the tests.

IMPORTANT APPLICATIONS OF DIRECT IMMUNOFLUORESCENCE TESTS IN CLINICAL AND PUBLIC HEALTH BACTERIOLOGY

In Table 1 are listed those applications of IF tests which: (a) are currently most common in clinical and public health laboratories, (b) appear to have high use potential, and (c) although they are excellent applications, find limited use due to the rarity of the disease concerned or because the reagents and experienced personnel required are not available. The tests are not listed in priority order. Comments on a few of them follow.

IF staining is used for serological grouping of Group A streptococci from hundreds of thousands of throat cultures each year in the U.S.A. The screening of foodstuffs and environmental specimens for the salmonellae by IF tests is growing rapidly, since satisfactory commercial reagents have become available. The procedure is undergoing extensive evaluation by the FDA and may soon be recommended for acceptance by the Association of Official Analytical Chemists (AOAC). Attempts have been made by Aerojet Medical and Biological Systems* to partially automate IF screening for the salmonellae. A slide processor similar to that used in the "seromatic" system for the indirect fluorescent-treponemal-antibody-absorbed (FTA-ABS) test was modified for single stage direct IF testing. An electronic slide reader scans

---

*Use of trade names is for identification only and does not constitute endorsement by the Public Health Service or by the U. S. Department of Health, Education, and Welfare.

Table 1. Status of immunofluorescence (IF) tests which are most useful in diagnostic bacteriology laboratories

Organism	Disease	Reported cases[a] (U.S.)	Status	Reference number
Direct IF tests				
1. Group A streptococci	Acute pharyngitis and scarlet fever	474,212	Most highly evaluated and most massively used of all IF tests for bacteria; sensitive and specific for detecting Group A streptococci from throat cultures.	1
	Acute rheumatic fever	2,560		
2. Group B streptococci	Neonatal meningitis and bovine mastitis		Polyvalent reagent containing both type and group antibody gave 99.1% agreement between IF and culture-precipitin tests on 833 clinical isolates and 97% agreement on 99 vaginal swabs; 8 false + reactions occurred in 982 clinical specimens; IF detected 9 nonhemolytic Group B's not detected by culture.	2
3. Serogrouping of enteropathogenic E. coli	Infant diarrhea	1,549 (15 states)	Highly effective for rapid screening of saline suspensions of feces. Eliminates culture of negatives.	1, 3
4. Salmonella typhosa	Typhoid fever	680	Vi conjugate equals culture for detection of chronic carriers. Make smears directly from saline suspension of feces. Less effective than culture for use on acute cases. Use OVi conjugate on smears of acute specimens prepared directly from saline suspension and from enrichments; also culture these specimens.	1, 4, 5

Continued.

Table 1. *Continued.*

Organism	Disease	Reported cases[a] (U.S.)	Status	Reference number
5. Salmonellae (most serotypes)	Gastroenteritis, enteric fever, meningitis	23,818 (Estimated 2 million cases/year)	Use a polyvalent conjugate covering "O" groups A-S to screen smears from tetrathionate or selenite enrichments of feces, foods, and environmental samples. Very sensitive but gives 1–20% IF positives on culture negative specimens. Culture all IF positives.	6–11
6. *Shigella* *S. sonnei*	Shigellosis	22,642	Sensitive and specific for screening saline suspensions of fecal smears. Well evaluated.	12, 13
S. flexneri			Appears promising for screening of fecal smears but needs further evaluation.	14, 15
7. *Bordetella pertussis* or *B. parapertussis*	Whooping cough	1,759	A rapid, sensitive, specific, and simple test for an organism for which culture is difficult. Stain pernasal-pharyngeal smears with specific conjugates.	1, 16, 17
8. Incitants of bacterial meningitis *H. influenzae* type b and/or types a–f	Do not use on throat smears.		These reagents when applied to CSF's are comparable in sensitivity to culture and Gram stain but are rapid, have immunological specificity, and will detect bacteria in partially treated patients. Superior for use on CSF's containing small numbers of organisms.	1, 18, 19

Organism	Disease	Number	Comments	References
Pneumococci	Do not use on throat smears.		Complex polyvalent conjugates needed for good coverage of capsular types (1–31); quite specific.	1, 18, 19
Meningococci (groups A–C)	Do not use on throat smears.	1,378	Polyvalent conjugate stains groups A and C well and group B less well. Also stains *N. gonorrhoeae.* May be used on smears from petechiae.	1, 18, 19
Listeria monocytogenes	Listeriosis	38 (14 states)	Excellent for specific detection of organisms in formalin-fixed, paraffin-embedded tissues, tissue imprints, body fluids, and cultures, including colonies from plates.	1
9. *Brucella suis, B. abortus, B. melitensis*	Brucellosis	202	Sensitive, rapid, and specific for smooth strains of these species in culture and tissues.	1
10. *Yersinia pestis*	Plague	2	Excellent for rapid diagnosis when used on blood, stored animal tissues, and stomach contents of vectors. Organisms stain well in tissue impression smears or in frozen or freeze-dried sections but not in routinely prepared formalin-fixed, paraffin-embedded sections. Conjugate is specific if carefully prepared or sorbed.	1
11. *Francisella tularensis*	Tularemia	171	Rapid, sensitive, and specific for detection of organisms in culture, impression smears and frozen or freeze-dried section of infected tissue specimens. Does not cross-stain *F. novicida* or *Brucella.* May stain *E. insidiosa* and a pseudomonad.	1

Continued.

Table 1. *Continued.*

Organism	Disease	Reported cases[a] (U.S.)	Status	Reference number
12. *Bacillus anthracis*	Anthrax	2	Rapid and sensitive for detection of anthrax organisms in culture, in tissue imprints, or in formalin-fixed, paraffin-embedded tissues of infected animals. Cross-stains some other species of bacilli.	1
13. *Mycobacterium tuberculosis*	Tuberculosis	31,015	Rapid and sensitive for detection of *M. tuberculosis* in direct sputum smears or digests; 98% of 96 culturally positive sputa were + by IF; 0 of 6 other mycobacterial species were +. Conjugates specific for *M. kansasii, M. phlei, M. marium,* and the u subgroup of Runyon's Group III have been prepared and tested.	20, 21
14. *Mycobacterium avium* complex	Swine, fowl, and human myco-bacterioses		Two pooled conjugates of 10 serotypes, which constitute 92% of the *M. avium* complex of organisms isolated from man, specifically stained homologous serotype cultures.	22
15. *Vibrio fetus* var. *venerealis*	Vibriosis		Reliable, simple, rapid means of diagnosing bovine vibriosis in the cow. Use filtered cervical-vaginal mucus. Does not differentiate *V. fetus* var. *venerealis* from *V. fetus* var. *intestinalis.*	23

Organism	Disease		Comments	Ref.
16. *Erysipelothrix insidiosa*	Infections in many animal species		Rapid, sensitive, and specific for detection of bacteria in cultures, blood, tissue imprints, and in histologically processed tissue sections. Labeled antibody to major shared antigens is used. Sensitivity compared to culture may be inadequate for routine diagnostic use on swine tissues.	24, 25
17. *Actinomyces* *A. israelii, A. naeslundii, A. eriksonii*	Actinomycosis		Rapid, sensitive, and specific for species (3) determination and for serotyping of *A. israelii* and *A. eriksonii* in pure or mixed cultures. Also useful with Gram staining for detecting organisms in human tonsils and other tissues or exudates.	26, 27
18. Clostridia *C. botulinum*	Botulism	34	Conjugates are available for differentiating toxin types A, B, and F from toxin types C and D, and from type E in cultures and in foods. Sensitive, rapid, and specific staining of bacteria in culture and in tissue imprints and sections, using a single "O" conjugate.	28, 29
C. chauvoei	Blackleg in cattle and other animals		Same as above when using a conjugate containing antibodies to the 2 "O" group antigens.	30
C. septicum	Braxy of sheep, malignant edema, gas gangrene		Same as above when using a single "O" conjugate.	30
C. novyi	Gas gangrene, necrotic hepatitis		Same as above when using a single "O" conjugate.	31
C. tetani	Tetanus	10	Same as above when using a single "O" conjugate.	31

Continued.

Table 1. *Continued.*

Organism	Disease	Reported cases[a] (U.S.)	Status	Reference number
19. *Leptospira* Multiple serotypes	Leptospirosis	57	Excellent for rapid and sensitive screening of formalin-preserved or fresh tissue scrapings or imprints and for cultures and urine sediments for the presence of pathogenic leptospires. Use a single group specific conjugate.	32
20. *Neisseria gonorrhoeae*	Gonorrhea	842,621	Usefulness limited to staining of organisms in pure culture, in conjunctivae, skin lesions and joint fluids, or for screening of mixed cultures for rapid presumptive information. Not recommended for diagnosis or for test of cure. Use only conjugates check tested for specificity by the CDC.	33
21. *Chlamydia trachomatis*	Trachoma	400–500 million (world) with 2 million totally blinded. Greatest single cause of preventable loss of vision (1973) (34)	IF is most sensitive method for detecting intracellular inclusions of the trachoma-inclusion conjunctivitis group of agents. It is highly specific.	34, 35
22. *Mycoplasma* sp.	Respiratory diseases, genital infections, and arthritis		Sensitive, rapid, and specific for detecting colonies by flooding plates with conjugate and observing by incident illumination.	36

		Incidence	Description	Reference
23. *Pseudomonas* *P. pseudomallei* *P. mallei*	Melioidosis Glanders		Rapid and sensitive for detecting bacteria in culture, exudates, and tissue imprints of infected animals. Conjugate for *P. pseudomallei* will also detect *P. mallei*. May cross-react with other pseudomonads.	37, 38
24. *T. pallidum*	Syphilis	87,469	Rapid procedure for detecting *Treponema pallidum* in early syphilitic lesions. Still experimental, but specificity appears adequate to differentiate saprophytic organisms in oral and rectal specimens from *T. pallidum.*	39
Indirect IF tests *T. pallidum*	Syphilis	87,469	FTA-ABS test should be used for verification and not for routine tests. Most sensitive of treponemal tests with specificity equal to the TPI. Not useful for evaluating therapeutic response. Recent data show that FTA-ABS tests for IgM antibody to *T. pallidum* in congenital infections may not be disease specific.	40-42

[a]Incidence data, except as noted, appeared in *Morbidity and Mortality Weekly Report*, No. 53, Vol. 22, for year ending December 29, 1973. U.S. Department of Health, Education, and Welfare, Public Health Service, Center for Disease Control, Atlanta, Georgia. Reprinted by permission.

the stained slide and records the fluorescence. These instruments have been evaluated both in the FDA and in our laboratory. Results at the CDC have been good with certain classes of food specimens but unsatisfactory with others. Both engineering and biological improvements are needed if the system is to gain acceptance in industrial or regulatory laboratories. Furthermore, it must be remembered that this system is based on the use of selective enrichments to permit multiplication of the salmonellae and synthesis of reactive surface antigens and to accomplish dilution of food substances which interfere with staining and interpretation of the IF reactions. The major biological problem arises from inability of the enrichment media to sustain selective multiplication of salmonellae when inoculated with specimens which are highly contaminated with other enteric bacterial flora.

The main advantage of the *Salmonella* detection procedure is its sensitivity and very low (1% or less) false negative rate. Thus, specimens which are negative by IF tests do not require plating and further study. IF positive samples must, however, be cultured and the salmonellae isolated and identified.

During 1974, our laboratory experienced a considerable increase in requests for assistance in the diagnosis of pertussis. This appears to reflect a real increase in pertussis or pertussis-like disease. Since many laboratories do not attempt the culture of *Bordetella pertussis* and *Bordetella parapertussis*, staining of pernasal-nasopharyngeal smears by specific conjugates for these organisms is very helpful in obtaining a diagnosis. Success depends upon obtaining an appropriate specimen during the first week of the disease and upon the availability of suitable IF reagents.

IF tests on cerebrospinal fluid (CSF) sediments in suspected cases of bacterial meningitis may contribute important guidance to the clinician in selecting a therapeutic agent. The major advantages of these tests are: (a) the bacteria are specifically stained in the CSF of partially treated patients who are culturally negative and (b) because of their sensitivity, IF tests frequently reveal small numbers of stained organisms which are not visualized by Gram-staining. This is especially important with Gram-negative bacteria.

IF tests are very important for detection of some of the rare but severe and life-threatening disease agents, such as *Yersinia pestis, Francisella tularensis, Bacillus anthracis,* and *Pseudomonas pseudomallei.* Unfortunately, satisfactory reagents are not usually available commercially, nor are personnel adequately experienced to interpret the results obtained. Thus, use of IF procedures as aids in the diagnosis of these unusual infections has been limited to a few specialty laboratories.

Although trachoma is not an important disease in the U. S. A., except among some Indians of the southwest, its causative agent was listed in Table 1 because of its global prevalence. The human misery and suffering plus the economic impact of two million people who have been completely blinded and tens of millions of others with seriously impaired vision as a result of this disease rank it high among the scourges of mankind. Trachoma is the greatest single cause of preventable loss of vision. Direct examination of conjunctival epithelial cells with an appropriate IF reagent is a very rapid, sensitive, and specific method of demonstrating the characteristic inclusion bodies of *Chlamydia trachomatis.*

AN IMPORTANT APPLICATION OF THE INDIRECT IF TEST IN THE CLINICAL AND PUBLIC HEALTH LABORATORY

The only indirect IF test for detecting bacterial antibody which is used routinely in many laboratories is the FTA-ABS test for syphilis. Not infrequently, however, the indirect test is used to detect various unknown antigens, thus avoiding the necessity of preparing specific conjugates for each of the antigenic species. For example, an antirabbit gamma globulin conjugate may be used to induce fluorescence of bacteria which have reacted with homologous antibacterial serum prepared by immunizing rabbits with the appropriate antigen. In this way, the necessity of preparing specific conjugates for each of the antigenic species is avoided. The disadvantages of this use are: (a) doubling of the staining period, (b) increased probability of nonspecific reactions, and (c) distortion of the morphology of the antigenic particles.

The FTA-ABS test has recently received undeserved criticism arising primarily from two areas. First, the specificity of the test has been questioned because some laboratories are using it for routine screening of sera, a purpose for which it was neither intended nor recommended. The result has been too many false positive tests, that is, positive FTA-ABS test results in sera from patients without a history or clinical evidence of syphilis. Other difficulties have arisen from the use of antihuman conjugates of inappropriate specificities. Second, problems inherent in the test itself, such as the nature of sorbent and the mechanism of its action, have not been resolved. As noted in discussing Table 1, recent data indicate that the FTA-ABS test modified for detection of IgM as an indication of congenital syphilis may not be disease specific (42). This difficulty stems from the production of rheumatoid factors (IgM-anti-IgG) in the sera of newborns and older persons.

NEEDS AND FUTURE DIRECTIONS OF IF TESTING IN BACTERIOLOGY LABORATORIES

Foremost among needs of the clinical and public health laboratories for improved IF testing is the provision of well-defined reagents of appropriate titer and specificity. Meeting these needs presupposes the existence of: (a) independent performance testing and evaluation capabilities, (b) acceptable standard testing procedures, and (c) appropriate reference reagents with which those under evaluation may be compared.

Insofar as the writer is aware, no responsible body has designated any bacterial conjugates for direct IF tests as official reference reagents. The same is true for the conjugates of antihuman immunoglobulins (Ig, IgG, IgM, and IgA), although valiant efforts are being made to prepare, evaluate, and obtain consensus on reagents which can be designated as national or international standards (43).

Quantitation of fluorescence measurements is an important aspect of IF standardization. The difficulties are great because of the unusually large number of variable factors requiring control. Fluorescence material standards, such as uranyl glass, phosphor crystals, or fluorescein solutions, are proving helpful in the measurement and standardization of fluorescence emission, but the most promising development is the use of insolubilized antigens to provide standards for more relevant immunological fluorescence comparisons (43, 44).

The physicochemical characterization of IF reagents is the obverse of the performance evaluation coin. When reagents are found to meet the required performance criteria in operational tests, their internal constitution is generally not closely scrutinized. When, however, the reagent fails to perform properly, the only hope for improvement lies in physicochemical analysis to identify and correct the deficiency. The important attributes of a conjugate are: (a) its content of specific antibody, (b) the relative content of immunoglobulins of the IgG and IgM classes, (c) the purity of the antibody-containing fraction, (d) the fluorescein-to-protein (F/P) (or fluorescein-to-antibody) ratio, and (e) the absence of free FITC.

Attributes b, c, d, and e above are relatively easy to determine for bacterial conjugates used in direct staining but a is more difficult to determine and, in practice, is usually not determined. Immunoelectrophoresis (CASE) furnished information on c, d, and e. The precise F/P ratio is calculated from data given by quantitative protein and fluorescein measurements. A useful manual for physiocochemical analysis of conjugates is that of Hebert et al. (45).

Another basic need closely related to progress in improving the performance of IF reagents is the provision of a pure preparation of FITC to serve as a standard reference material. Only adequate sponsorship and modest funds are required to achieve this goal because the technology is available.

Finally, improvements are being made in fluorescence microscopy, the most important being the introduction of incident or epi-illumination. The combination of incident illumination, halogen lamps, and interference filters for excitation has resulted in simpler and relatively less expensive, but generally satisfactory, viewing systems.

As the technology improves and reagents of high quality become more readily available, IF techniques will find an expanding role in clinical and public health bacteriology laboratories.

LITERATURE CITED

1. Cherry, W. B., and M. D. Moody. 1965. Fluorescent-antibody techniques in diagnostic bacteriology. Bact. Rev. 29:222–250.

2. Romero, R., and H. W. Wilkinson. 1974. Identification of Group B streptococci by immunofluorescence staining. Appl. Microbiol. 28:199–204.

3. Thomason, B. M., and W. B. Cherry. 1971. Misuse of fluorescent antibody tests for detection of enteropathogenic *Escherichia coli*. Am. J. Med. Tech. 37(6):258–259.

4. Thomason, B. M., and A. C. McWhorter. 1965. Rapid detection of typhoid carriers by means of fluorescent antibody techniques. Bull. World Health Organ. 33:681–685.

5. Bissett, M. L., C. Powers, and R. M. Wood. 1969. Immunofluorescent identification of *Salmonella typhi* during a typhoid outbreak. Appl. Microbiol. 17:507–511.

6. Thomason, B. M., and J. G. Wells. 1971. Preparation and testing of polyvalent conjugates for fluorescent-antibody detection of salmonellae. Appl. Microbiol. 22:876–884.

7. Thomason, B. M., and G. A. Hebert. 1974. Evaluation of commercial conjugates for fluorescent antibody detection of salmonellae. Appl. Microbiol. 27:862–869.

8. Demissie, A. 1966. Studies on epidemiological salmonellosis by fluorescent antibody technique. Acta. path. et microbiol. scandiv. 67:393–400.

9. Stulberg, C. S., W. J. Caldwell, D. W. Kennedy, and G. Caldroney. 1966. Epidemiologic and diagnostic application of immunofluorescence in a *Salmonella* outbreak. J. Epidemiol. 83:518–529.

10. Mohr, H. K., H. L. Trenk, and M. Yeterian. 1974. Comparison of fluorescent-antibody methods and enrichment serology for the detection of *Salmonella*. Appl. Microbiol. 27:324–328.

11. Insalata, N. F., W. G. Dunlap, and C. W. Mahnke. 1973. Evaluation of the *Salmonella* fluoro-kit for fluorescent antibody staining. Appl. Microbiol. 25:202–204.

12. Taylor, C. E. D., G. V. Heimer, D. J. Lea, and A. J. H. Tomlinson. 1964. A comparison of a fluorescent antibody technique with a cultural method in the detection of infections with *Shigella sonnei*. J. Clin. Path. 17:225–230.

13. Taylor, C. E. D., and G. V. Heimer. 1964. Rapid diagnosis of Sonne dysentery by means of immunofluorescence. Brit. M. J. 2:165–166.

14. Thomason, B. M., G. S. Cowart, and W. B. Cherry. 1965. Current status of immunofluorescence techniques for rapid detection of shigellae in fecal specimens. Appl. Microbiol. 13:605–613.

15. Thomason, B. M., A. J. Nahmias, and A. D. Mathews. 1967. Further evaluation of immunofluorescence techniques for detection of shigellae in fecal specimens. Appl. Microbiol. 15:912–915.

16. Whitaker, J. A., P. Donaldson, and J. D. Nelson. 1960. Diagnosis of pertussis by the fluorescent-antibody method. New England J. Med. 263:850–851.

17. Pittman, B. 1974. *Bordetella. In* E. H. Lennette, E. H. Spaulding, and J. P. Truant (eds.), Manual of Clinical Microbiology, Ed. 2, pp. 308–315. American Society for Microbiology, Washington, D.C.

18. Biegeleisen, J. Z., Jr., M. S. Mitchell, B. B. Marcus, D. L. Rhoden, and R. W. Blumberg. 1965. Immunofluorescence techniques for demonstrating bacterial pathogens associated with cerebrospinal meningitis. I. Clinical

evaluation of conjugates on smears prepared directly from cerebrospinal fluid sediments. J. Lab. & Clin. Med. 65:976–989.

19. Fox, H. A., P. A. Hagen, D. J. Turner, L. A. Glasgow, and J. D. Connor. 1969. Immunofluorescence in the diagnosis of acute bacterial meningitis: A cooperative evaluation of the technique in a clinical laboratory setting. Pediatrics 43:44–49.

20. Jones, W. D., R. E. Beam, and G. P. Kubica. 1966. Fluorescent antibody techniques with mycobacteria. II. Detection of *Mycobacterium tuberculosis* in sputum. Am. Rev. Resp. Dis. 95:516–517.

21. Jones, W. D., Jr., and G. P. Kubica. 1968. Fluorescent antibody techniques with mycobacteria. III. Investigation of five serologically homogeneous groups of mycobacteria. Zentralbl. Bakt. (Abt. I Orig.) 175:582–604.

22. Gales, P. W., R. R. Martins, and W. E. Walker. 1974. Production of multivalent fluorescent antisera for identification of organisms in the *Mycobacterium avium-Mycobacterium intracellulare* complex. Appl. Microbiol. 27:753–755.

23. Shires, G. M. H., and T. T. Kramer. 1974. Filtration of bovine cervicovaginal mucus for diagnosis of vibriosis, using the fluorescent antibody test. J. Am. Vet. M. A. 164:398–401.

24. Marshall, J. D., W. C. Eveland, and C. W. Smith. 1959. The identification of viable and nonviable *Erysipelothrix insidiosa* with fluorescent antibody. Am. J. Vet. Res. 20:1077–1080.

25. Harrington, R., Jr., and R. L. Wood. 1974. Comparison of fluorescent antibody technique and cultural method for the detection of *Erysipelothrix rhusiopathiae* in primary broth cultures. Am. J. Vet. Res. 35:461–462.

26. Blank, C. H., and L. K. Georg. 1968. The use of fluorescent antibody methods for the detection and identification of *Actinomyces* species in clinical material. J. Lab. & Clin. Med. 71:283–293.

27. Brock, D. W., and L. K. Georg. 1969. Determination and analysis of *Actinomyces israelii* serotypes by fluorescent-antibody procedures. J. Bact. 97:581–588.

28. Walker, P. D., and I. Batty. 1964. Fluorescent studies in the genus *Clostridium*. II. A rapid method for differentiating *Clostridium botulinum* types A, B and F, types C and D, and type E. J. Appl. Bact. 27:140–142.

29. Midura, T. F., Y. Inouye, and H. L. Bodily. 1967. Use of immunofluorescence to identify *Clostridium botulinum* Types A, B, and E. Pub. Health Rep. 82:275–279.

30. Batty, I., and P. D. Walker. 1963. Fluorescent labelled clostridial antisera as specific stains. Bull. Office Int. Epizoot. 59:1499–1513.

31. Batty, I., and P. D. Walker. 1964. The identification of *Clostridium novyi (Clostridium oedematiens)* and *Clostridium tetani* by the use of fluorescent labelled antibodies. J. Path. & Bact. 88:327–328.

32. Maestrone, G. 1963. The use of an improved fluorescent antibody procedure in the demonstration of leptospira in animal tissues. Canad. J. Comp. Med. Vet. Sc. 27:108–112.

33. U. S. Department of Health, Education, and Welfare. 1972. Criteria and techniques for the diagnosis of gonorrhea. Public Health Service, CDC, Atlanta.

34. Field methods for the control of trachoma. 1973. M. L. Tarizzo (ed.), World Health Organization, Geneva.

35. Hanna, L., J. Schachter, and E. Jawetz. 1974. Chlamydiae (Psittacosis-lymphogranuloma venereum-trachoma group). *In* E. H. Lennette, E. H.

Spaulding, and J. P. Truant (eds.), Manual of Clinical Microbiology, Ed. 2, pp. 795–804. American Society for Microbiology, Washington, D.C.

36. Del Giudice, R. A., M. F. Robillard, and T. R. Carski. 1967. Immunofluorescence identification of *Mycoplasma* on agar by use of incident illumination. J. Bact. 93:1205–1209.

37. Moody, M. D., M. Goldman, and B. M. Thomason. 1956. Staining bacterial smears with fluorescent antibody. I. General methods for *Malleomyces pseudomallei*. J. Bact. 72:357–361.

38. Thomason, B. M., M. D. Moody, and M. Goldman. 1956. Staining bacterial smears with fluorescent antibody. II. Rapid detection of varying numbers of *Malleomyces pseudomallei* in contaminated materials and infected animals. J. Bact. 72:362–367.

39. Wallace, A. L., and L. C. Norins. 1969. Syphilis serology today. Prog. Clin. Path. 11:198–215.

40. U. S. Department of Health, Education, and Welfare. 1969. Manual of tests for syphilis. Public Health Service Publication No. 411 (Revised), U. S. Government Printing Office, Washington.

41. U. S. Department of Health, Education, and Welfare. 1971. The laboratory aspects of syphilis. Public Health Service, CDC, Atlanta.

42. Reimer, C. B., C. M. Black, D. J. Phillips, L. C. Logan, E. F. Hunter, B. J. Pender, and B. E. McGrew. 1975. The specificity of fetal IgM: Antibody or anti-antibody? Ann. N. Y. Acad. Sci. 254:77–93.

43. Cherry, W. B., and C. B. Reimer. 1973. Diagnostic immunofluorescence. Bull. World Health Organ. 48:737–746.

44. Dalen, J. P. R. van, W. Knapp, and J. S. Ploem. 1973. Microfluorimetry on antigen-antibody interaction in immunofluorescence using antigens covalently bound to agarose beads. J. Immun. Meth. 2:383–392.

45. Hebert, G. A., B. Pittman, R. M. McKinney, and W. B. Cherry. 1972. The preparation and physicochemical characterization of fluorescent antibody reagents. U. S. Department of Health, Education, and Welfare, Public Health Service, CDC, Atlanta.

CHAPTER 7

Systems for the Isolation and Identification of Anaerobic Bacteria

Genevieve S. Nygaard

It can be accurately assumed that the methods used to routinely handle any bacteria will result in trauma to the organism. Organisms may be traumatized during collection of a sample as well as during its transportation to the laboratory. In the laboratory are added the insults of stale or overcooked food (frequently offered only after much delay) along with temperatures that may fluctuate rapidly from too low to too high. Additionally, in dealing with anaerobic bacteria, there is the insult of exposure to atmosphere which contains the toxic gas, oxygen. Any bacteriologist knows that maximum growth of bacteria can be expected only when all their growth demands are met optimally, and that, conversely, varying from optimum conditions will decrease the volume of growth and even result in death of the bacteria. Anaerobic bacteriological work simply tests our willingness and ability to actively apply this knowledge.

COLLECTION AND TRANSPORTATION

Collection and transportation of specimens is important in any area of bacteriology and is of paramount importance in anaerobic bacteriology. This subject has been discussed in detail by many workers (1–3). Results of their findings should be carefully studied and implemented since this phase is vital to the success of subsequent laboratory examinations. A large percentage of samples which should be routinely cultured for anaerobic bacteria are, or can be, obtained by aspiration (4). Aspirated material in a closed syringe is, in essence, in an anaerobic chamber. Closing off the end of the needle still attached to the syringe by inserting it into a hard stopper allows the specimen to be safely transported limited distances to the laboratory. The aspirate can be transferred through a rubber closure into a sterile vial or bottle containing oxygen-free gas. Before doing this, a small amount of specimen should be ejected through the needle and discarded in order to clear the needle of air and to prevent the introduction of oxygen into the vial with the sample. Biopsy samples can also be placed in gassed bottles by opening and inserting the sample as quickly as possible. Entrance of air cannot be avoided under these circumstances unless a gassing cannula (Figure 1) is used, but the anaerobes will be protected for a time as a result of the continued respiration of the tissue itself. Swab samples should be strongly discouraged. If it is necessary to collect a specimen by this means, specially prepared sterilized swabs held in tubes containing oxygen-free gas must be used and the swab must then be placed in a second tube also containing oxygen-free gas. As with the biopsy samples, some air will be introduced unless a gassing cannula is used. Some workers favor use of semisolid holding medium to an empty tube. The holding medium protects the sample more effectively from exposure to oxygen but may dilute it mechanically. While the empty tube does not dilute the sample, it does allow for greater exposure to the oxygen introduced. The best solution is to avoid, whenever possible, use of swabs as a means of collecting specimens for detection of anaerobic bacteria.

ISOLATION METHODS

Exclusion or protection from oxygen when handling anaerobes is the single major problem that differs from those that must be dealt with in connection

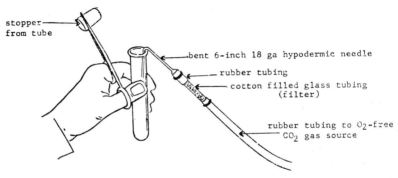

stopper from tube

bent 6-inch 18 ga hypodermic needle

rubber tubing

cotton filled glass tubing (filter)

rubber tubing to O_2-free CO_2 gas source

Figure 1. Gassing cannula. (From Holdeman and Moore (2). With permission of authors.)

with isolation of aerobes. Such exclusion can most effectively be accomplished in the laboratory through the use of a closed system from which oxygen has been removed and which prevents the re-entry of this gas at all stages of processing. There are essentially two major systems that have been successfully used to accomplish this. One utilizes individual tubes containing pre-reduced anaerobically sterilized (PRAS) media and is commonly spoken of as the roll-tube method (2, 3, 5–7). The second employs an anaerobic chamber or glove-box (2, 3, 6, 8, 9). These systems undoubtedly allow for the most ideal handling of anaerobic bacteria.

The individual or roll-tube system requires the least initial cost and the least space. Minimum components needed if this system is used are: (a) a tank of compressed gas, (b) a gas regulator with a needle valve control, (c) a gassing cannula which is essentially a large bent hypodermic needle, (d) supports (such as a ring stand with clamps for these last two items), (e) forceps for removing and replacing the stoppers from the PRAS media tubes, and (f) a tube rotator. A more sophisticated form of this inoculation and transfer system is the V.P.I. Inoculator* (Bellco Glass, Inc.) which provides two additional cannulas, tube holders and foot pedal controls (Figure 2), all of which permit easier manipulation of additional tubes as well as multiple transfer possibilities. While such a unit may appear difficult to operate, the learning time necessary for a microbiologist to acquire reasonable proficiency is less than half a day. The equivalent of a 20-in deep by 54-in length bench space will accommodate such a unit along with the supportive compressed gas tank. This space allows for the inoculator itself plus a burner, rack of tubes, pipette discard jar, and small tools (such as loops, forceps, etc.) needed during operations.

PRAS media is commercially available from only one company (Scott Laboratories) at the present time. The cost per tube (about $0.45–$0.50) is approximately two to three times what one probably pays for media used in the isolation and identification of aerobes. Shelf-life is at least 3 months from the date of preparation but has been reported to be as long as a year or more (W. E. C. Moore, unpublished data). Tubes of PRAS can be incubated in racks in any incubator. They can be opened, using the gassing cannula, at any time without disturbing growth of the culture if it is desirable to remove an aliquot for making smears or for any other reason. Streaked roll-tubes can be observed using magnification, such as a dissecting or stereoscope to distinguish colony types, and to make pickings from growth at any time without loss of anaerobic conditions. The strongest objections that have been raised to the use of this method is that in roll-streak tubes it is difficult to distinguish and to pick individual colonies. Fifteen-millimeter-diameter tubes originally used tested one's steadiness of hand; currently used 25-mm tubes are not as much of a problem in this respect and allow a greater surface area for

---

*Use of trade names is for purposes of identification and does not imply endorsement by the California Department of Health.

V.P.I. ANAEROBIC CULTURE SYSTEM (Bellco, Inc.)

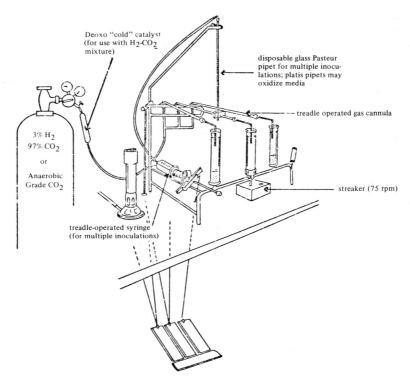

Figure 2. V.P.I. inoculator. (From Holdeman and Moore (2). With permission of authors.)

isolation. Use of the dissecting microscope, however, is a technique which should be strongly recommended for use both with surface streaked plates as well as with roll-tubes.

Anaerobic chambers vary markedly in size and in structure. Primarily there are the soft versus the rigid-walled types. One soft-walled unit (Figure 3) produced commercially (Coy Manufacturing Co.) has one pair of gloves and fits on a table top 39-in deep by 99-in in length; these dimensions include a 22-in length under the entry-lock through which materials must be passed in and out of the chamber. A larger version, which has two pairs of gloves, requires a 39-in by 118-in space; again this includes a 22-in length under the entry-lock. This larger chamber allows for placement of a small incubator inside. If an internal incubator is not included, then inoculated media is placed in anaerobe jars which are removed from the chamber for incubation. The chamber system also requires compressed gas with regulator and flow controls, catalyst pellets, heater unit to dry the pellets, and an electric

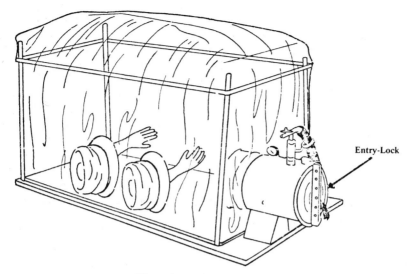

Figure 3. Anaerobe chamber.

inoculating-loop sterilizer. Freshly prepared media can be introduced into the chamber and stored there prior to use to allow for the development of satisfactory redox levels. Plates can be surface streaked and tubed media can be inoculated in the manner one is accustomed to on the open bench. However, training or adjustment time is necessary because the wearing of medium weight gloves reduces tactile sense and one's area of operation is limited by the porthole arrangement. Incorporation of an incubator within the unit allows for observations to be made at any time just as with roll-streak tubes. Magnification is strongly recommended for these procedures. It is possible to seal a dissecting microscope into the soft- and even the rigid-walled chamber so that such observations can be most effectively carried out. The chief advantage of this system is that inoculation of plates and tubes can be carried on in essentially the same manner one uses in working with aerobic bacteria. Also, as with the roll-streak method, rapidity of observations and transfer procedures is not critical because the bacteria are held in an anaerobic atmosphere. The primary disadvantages are the space requirements, time lost in having to pass through the entry-lock all items added to or removed from the chamber, and the initial cost (Coy's basic small chamber will cost approximately four times that of one V.P.I. Inoculator).

As stated earlier, these two systems, V.P.I. Inoculator and anaerobic chamber, undoubtedly allow for the most ideal handling of anaerobic bacteria. Some bacteriologists believe that they are not necessary because the very sensitive anaerobes, which can only be isolated under such conditions, are not known to be involved in infectious processes in man. It is readily apparent that this could be a self-perpetuating concept: one does not use such techniques because they are not needed; therefore, the organisms requiring such techniques are not isolated, and so, such techniques are not needed, ad infinitum. Comparative studies that have already been carried out using optimum methods support the concept that the most sensitive types of anaerobes are either not involved in infections in man or are very rarely involved (9–11). A more valid argument for use of the best techniques possibly is the concept that small numbers of organisms and environmentally debilitated organisms will be more readily and rapidly detected in the presence of optimal growth conditions. The method used in the collection and transportation of the specimen to the laboratory may already have subjected the organism(s) to extremely adverse conditions. Therefore, use of optimal procedures once the specimen is received in the laboratory becomes even more essential. This concept applies to the more hardy of the anaerobic organisms as well as to those very fastidious ones. Application of improved techniques already has moved the subject from an era when reported anaerobic infections were almost entirely limited to gas gangrene and tetanus to the present when reports of infections in which anaerobes are known to be involved include most tissues and cavities of the body (4, 12–19). Whether we now have a full measure of the infectious ability of this group of organisms is as yet unknown.

A less complex method that has shown highly satisfactory results is open bench top plating followed by incubation in anaerobe jars. Anaerobic conditions are developed within the jar through replacement of the gasses within the jar or through generation of gasses from chemicals placed in the jar. Use of these jars is probably familiar to most microbiologists. Satisfactory results, however, depend upon the proper use of this equipment with attention to a number of details. Many references call attention to the need for heating the palladium-coated catalyst pellets between each use in order to prevent loss of activity (3, 6, 7, 10). While removal of oxygen from the jar's atmosphere is dependent upon its combination with hydrogen, increased amounts of carbon dioxide should also be incorporated into the jar for maximum growth (20). Insertion of a methylene blue indicator into a jar each time it is used will help to control proper atmospheric conditions. Another factor, which has been repeatedly commented upon, is that anaerobe jars should routinely *not* be opened before a 48-hr incubation period has been allowed (2, 7, 9, 16, 20). At the end of the 18- to 24-hr incubation period, when these jars are frequently opened, most anaerobic growth will not yet be visible. Anaerobes which have recovered enough to be starting out of their lag phase and are beginning to climb up the slope of the growth curve are due for a setback as a result of the exposure to oxygen. Such exposure may terminate the culture. The only safe procedure for satisfactory work, when a jar must be opened before 48 hrs, is to have duplicate sets of plates placed in separate jars. One jar may then be opened as early as desired and the second jar held for a more satisfactory 48- to 72-hr incubation period.

No matter when the anaerobe jar is opened, the growth on the plates can be better protected if some type of purge- or flow-through jar (Figure 4), such as suggested by Martin (21), is employed to hold the plates, and they are then removed one at a time for necessary observations and picking. A variety of gasses can be used to pass through such jars to maintain a more suitable environment for the anaerobes: anaerobic grade carbon dioxide, 3% hydrogen with the balance carbon dioxide, or 10% carbon dioxide with 10% hydrogen and the balance nitrogen. The latter two combinations should be passed through a deoxo cold catalyst cartridge for removal of trace amounts of oxygen. A freshly boiled tube of methylene blue indicator can be inserted in the purge-jar each day to provide a check of the general level of anaerobiosis present. Such purge-jars can be used most advantageously to store freshly prepared plates prior to and after inoculation until they can be placed under better anaerobic conditions.

One of the major disadvantages of the anaerobe jar system handled on the bench top, as opposed to setting it up and opening it within an anaerobe

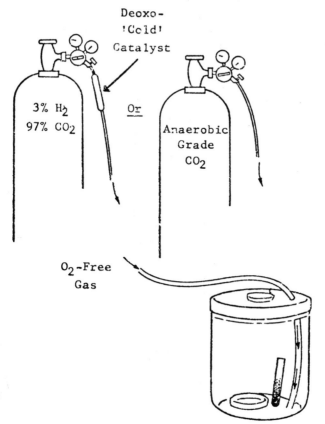

Figure 4. Purge-jar system. (From Martin (21). With permission of author.)

chamber, is the need for duplication of plating. Double jars mean double initial cost of this equipment. At present, the purchase price of two anaerobe jars is slightly more than half the cost of one V.P.I. inoculator. More importantly, it means markedly increased work due to double planting procedures, observations, and all other steps. Also, the organisms one is attempting to grow are unavoidably exposed to oxygen.

One need not use one method to the exclusion of the other. Many laboratories have found that a combination of systems best answers their needs. Undoubtedly a large number of laboratories either use or will choose to use the anaerobe jar method. If this is the method selected, then the purge- or flow-through jar support system used as an adjunct, is strongly recommended (2, 16). Both its use and practicality have been tested. Once one has compressed gas available to him, it is relatively easy to add a gassing cannula and a motor driven unit (Figure 5) for inoculating roll-streak tubes or inoculating other PRAS media tubes. These roll-streak tubes can profitably serve as backup tubes to be used if one's jars fail due to leakage, etc., or if one fails to isolate those organisms which appear to be present. Experience in our laboratory supports reports such as Malone's (unpublished) at the 1973 National American Public Health Association Meeting that such combinations of techniques are both practical and useful.

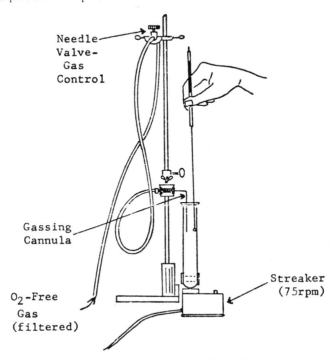

Needle—
Valve-
Gas
Control

Gassing
Cannula

O_2-Free
Gas
(filtered)

Streaker
(75rpm)

Figure 5. Gassing cannula and streaker.

PRIMARY HANDLING AND BIOCHEMICAL TESTING

A basic step in any protocol should be to make preparations for microscopic examinations from all specimens (with the exception of bloods). Stained and wet mount preparations should be carefully and thoroughly examined in order to alert the microbiologist to the presence of organisms and their relative numbers. Quite frankly, most bacteriologists have not been trained to carry out this step in a really satisfactory manner. If it had been performed properly more often in the past, there should have been far more questions raised as to why so many specimens from reportedly sterile abscesses clearly contained bacteria in their microscopic preparations.

The next step is to directly culture from the specimen to a general support medium in a manner which will allow for isolation of single colony growth. Media used in anaerobic culturing is not only important from a nutritional point of view, but many of the ingredients, such as cysteine hydrochloride, sodium sulfide, thioglycollate, metallic iron, and fragments of chopped meat, are important in maintenance of an adequate oxidation-reduction potential (7, 20). Some of these reducing agents can form toxic compounds when combined with oxygen and should be added to the media only after removal of as much oxygen as possible. In addition, some materials added to the media serve to neutralize toxic substances, which are correctly or incorrectly called "organic peroxides," and which develop as a result of exposure to oxygen, heat, light, and other factors; examples of these neutralizing compounds are starch, blood, and serum. Naturally, methods of preparation and storage which avoid the development of such toxic substances are advisable.

Most bacteriologists now supplement their base media, such as peptone-yeast or brain heart infusion, with vitamin K (or menadione) and hemin to permit or enchance the growth of commonly encountered species. A number of other substances, bile, tween, and various carbohydrates, also act to enhance the growth of different species or strains, and laked blood is commonly used to speed up and enhance pigment production of *Bacteroides melaninogenicus.*

While all specimens should be placed on general support media, selective media, which may prevent overgrowth by spreaders or more hardy growers, can also be used effectively both for primary isolation and for presumptive identification or grouping (22–25). Some of the compounds most commonly used, singly or in combinations, are phenylethyl alcohol, neomycin, vancomycin, and kanamycin.

As soon as it is possible to pick from single colonies, such transfers should be made to a general support broth such as chopped meat glucose, brain heart infusion supplemented with vitamin K and hemin, or thioglycollate glucose supplemented with vitamin K and hemin as well as with Filde's extract and sodium bicarbonate (2, 3). Stained smears should be prepared from the

colony and aerotolerance tests set up. Checking this characteristic is important even though no growth is noted on duplicate cultures made from the
clinical sample and incubated under carbon dioxide or aerobically. Facultative organisms sometimes fail to grow except under anaerobic conditions on
primary isolation.

One of the simplest procedures which provides much added information,
and one which may be required for accurate identification, is determination
of metabolical products by chromotography; typically, gas-liquid chromotography (2, 3, 6, 26). This procedure not only assists in making correct
identifications but also can provide results which will indicate errors in
presumptive identification, such as mistaking propionic producing bacteria
for *Actinomyces species,* or *Clostridium ramosum,* an easily decolorized
species which may not sporulate well, for a member of the Bacteroidaceae
family. The technique is simple and the equipment is relatively inexpensive;
currently, costs for a suitable chromatograph plus a recorder will range from
just under $2,000 to about $3,500. Tests can usually be carried out on 24- to
48-hr growth in carbohydrate broth. Extraction time plus instrument time
varies from ½ hr to probably a maximum of 1½ hr, depending on the number
of products of the isolate and on some slight variations in the extraction
procedures.

Additional cultural characteristics and biochemical test results, when
added to the chromatographic findings, will allow definitive identification.
Which particular tests should be performed can be found in a number of
manuals. Three manuals which any laboratory will find useful are those of:
(a) the Center for Disease Control, (b) the Veterans' Administration, Wads-
worth Hospital Center, and (c) the Virginia Polytechnic Institute (V.P.I.)
and State University. While each of these manuals contains much of the same
general and basic information, each offers a slightly different approach or
point of view and contains material that most laboratories will find useful.
The CDC manual is well organized and is easy to follow as a result of this and
the size type that has been used. It will be found particularly useful in
relation to toxin testing and to food examinations, subjects not specifically
covered or not covered in as much detail in the other two manuals. Finegold's
group at the Veterans' Administration Hospital emphasizes the clinical background of anaerobic infections and utilizes selective techniques, along with
other limited tests, for presumptive grouping or presumptive identification of
isolates. The single most complete listing of anaerobic bacteria, along with
their biochemical reaction patterns, chromatograms, etc., is contained in the
V.P.I. manual. The keys in this manual are unfamiliar to many, but can be
quickly learned. They are unusually compact, as is the entire manual. When
using any identification keys, variation in method and/or criteria of reading
may result in discrepancies in results.

While the quality of the base medium used, and the care taken to protect
the organisms from exposure to oxygen, is less critical when performing

biochemical tests because massive inoculums are characteristically used, these factors are still important for the most rapid and accurate results. In performing biochemical tests, some laboratories may find it most practical to use the same media used in their aerobic work. If this medium is (or is similar to) phenol red broth, it should be placed in a boiling water bath before inoculation to drive off the oxygen, and then detoxified and enriched through the addition of rabbit serum (final serum concentration about 10%). Using this procedure, satisfactory results can be obtained with many anaerobic bacteria when these biochemical tests are incubated in anaerobe jars. Thioglycollate broth without indicator can likewise be used, after heating in a boiling bath, as a base medium for biochemical testing but without the necessity of incubation in an anaerobe jar. Addition of serum may be necessary. Readings of pH changes with both these methods require the addition of an indicator following incubation because of the reduction of all pH indicators under anaerobic conditions. If an anaerobic chamber is available, these types of media can be stored in the chamber for 24 to 48 hr prior to inoculation to obtain satisfactory oxidation-reduction potentials and avoid the boiling water-bath step. Without prior heating, PRAS media in tubes can be inoculated on the open bench using the gassing cannula to exclude oxygen and can then be incubated in the aerobic incubator. With this media, determination of pH changes is based on pH meter readings, which results in objective readings rather than the more subjective readings that come from indicator dyes. This latter system permits the identification of even the most sensitive anaerobes. While the other biochemical testing methods do not allow for satisfactory work with as many anaerobes, they give satisfactory results with the most commonly isolated ones. When they are used, more frequent referral of isolates to reference laboratories is indicated.

Several kit-type systems have been and are being developed for use with anaerobic bacteria. While some of these have received field testing, very few reports have as yet appeared in the scientific literature (27, 28). Two of these kit systems, the API system from Analytab Products, Inc. and the Minitek system from BioQuest, with which our laboratory has had some limited experience, can be briefly discussed as examples.

The API system comes as a strip with fixed number and types of tests to be performed, while the Minitek system uses individual discs and, thus, allows each laboratory to select the tests to be done. An individual API strip costs just under $3.00 at present; the same number of examinations performed by the Minitek method will be approximately the same cost. The expiration date on an unopened API strip will be a maximum of 1 year. Once opened, a vial of Minitek discs has a shelf-life of 2 months no matter what the expiration date of the unopened vial. Basic hardware for the Minitek method costs about $300.00, while no special hardware is needed with the API strips; both systems require incubation in anaerobe jars; either would be most ideally handled in an anaerobic chamber for inoculation and incubation since this would allow the maximum protection of the organisms from adverse conditions during inoculum preparation and transfers. (The micro nature of these methods increases the importance of this factor.) Incubation in an anaerobic chamber would also make it possible to observe changes at intervals rather than only after 48 hr, which is the described incubation time in the anaerobe jars for both systems. If one accepts literally the use of the color-chip reading guide provided by BioQuest to decide on positive and negative reactions, an unacceptable number of errors can result. While experienced workers will probably adjust and set up their own reading scale, the inexperienced person should be wary.

To date, far more data has been accumulated on the results that can be expected from a variety of species and strains of anaerobes tested in the API system. Limited experience (unpublished) in our laboratory, however, has indicated that, when the results of the API kit were supplemented only by microscopic observations and the API key was used, not more than 70% of the isolates tested could be correctly identified. These figures correspond rather closely with the 66% correct identifications reported by Starr et al. (27). When additional tests, including gas-liquid chromotography, are performed, the accuracy of identification can be markedly improved, but other keys must then be used. Since the agreement between individual test results obtained in the API system and those obtained by other methods (PRAS, CDC thio-technique, etc.) is reported to be around 90%, it appears that the primary need is for improvements within the API keys for identification (26, 27). This could automatically come about as additional data is accumulated and integrated into the system.

Results obtained with the Minitek system in our limited studies (unpublished) are similar to those obtained with the API system: agreement of individual test results is around 90%. When the Minitek results alone are used along with the keys provided, only 65 to 70% of the organisms could be correctly identified. Inclusion of additional tests, such as gas-liquid chromotography, increased the accuracy of identification; other keys, of course, had to be employed.

Further evaluations of both systems are needed, especially with clinical isolates, to determine and clearly define the applications and limitations of these systems.

ANTIBIOTIC SUSCEPTIBILITY TESTING

One of the final procedures that requires consideration in a clinical laboratory performing anaerobic bacteriology is that of antibiotic susceptibility testing. All of the factors which influence results in susceptibility tests performed with aerobic bacteria are equally applicable when working with anaerobic bacteria. Other factors, such as effect of carbon dioxide in the atmosphere on the aminoglycosides and the effect of varying growth rates, etc., are important and influence test results (29–37). Experts across the country are presently collaborating in comparisons of methods with the goal of establishing a standard method.

In the meantime, one may select from a variety of published techniques. No matter which method is selected, one must adhere carefully to the established protocol if the author's reading standards are to be used and if useful information is to be made available to the clinician and to other workers in the field.

Use of discs has been described in connection with both agar and broth techniques (2, 3, 33, 35–37). The disc-agar diffusion methods have been most useful and reliable with rapid growers, while the broth-disc method has been successfully applied also to slower growing and more fastidious strains. Broth and agar techniques have also been described to establish minimum inhibitory concentrations (3, 38) or to establish a categorization system as reported by Stalons, Thornsberry, and Balows (39).

A number of studies have supplied information on the most effective current treatment for infections with a variety of anaerobic species (4, 14, 32, 38, 40–43). Many will prefer to use this information in place of obtaining susceptibility results on some isolates which are made; in the face of the technical difficulties and the problems associated with the interpretation of test results, authorities in this field tend to discourage routine susceptibility testing of anaerobic organisms. When susceptibility testing is required, it is suggested that full and complete perusal of the available literature be made and the results analyzed on the basis of knowledge regarding the limitations of the procedures used.

This presentation has not been an attempt to detail methods for anaerobic bacteriology. Rather, it has been an attempt to call attention to and briefly discuss the various factors that are involved in, and must be considered, when selecting the methods and protocols that will meet individual objectives and conditions, albeit with limitations that are recognized and can be accepted.

LITERATURE CITED

1. Dowell, Jr., V. R. 1974. Collection of clinical specimens and primary isolation of anaerobic bacteria. *In* A. Balows, R. M. Dehaan, V. R. Dowell, Jr., and L. B. Guze (eds.), Anaerobic Bacteria: Role in Disease, pp. 9–20. Charles C Thomas, Publisher, Springfield, Ill.

2. Holdeman, L. V., and W. E. C. Moore. 1972. Anaerobe Laboratory Manual. V.P.I. Anaerobe Laboratory, Virginia Polytechnic Institute, State University, Blacksburg, Virginia.

3. Sutter, V. L., H. R. Attebery, J. E. Rosenblatt, K. S. Bricknell, and S. M. Finegold. 1972. Anaerobic Bacteriology Manual. Department of Continuing

Education in Health Sciences, University Extension, and The School of Medicine of The University of California at Los Angeles, Los Angeles, Calif.

4. Finegold, S. M., J. E. Rosenblatt, V. L. Sutter, and H. R. Attebery. 1972. Scope Monograph on Anaerobic Infections. The Upjohn Company, Kalamazoo, Mich.
5. Crawford, J. M., J. R. Sconyers, J. M. Moriarty, R. C. King, and J. F. West. 1974. Bacteremia after tooth extractions studied with the aid of prereduced anaerobically sterilized media. Appl. Microbiol. 27:927–932.
6. Dowell, Jr. V. R., and T. M. Hawkins. 1974. Laboratory Methods in Anaerobic Bacteriology: CDC Laboratory Manual. U. S. Department of Health, Education and Welfare, Public Health Service, Center for Disease Control, Atlanta, Ga.
7. Smith, L. D. S., and L. V. Holdeman. 1968. The Pathogenic Anaerobic Bacteria. Charles C Thomas, Publisher, Springfield, Ill.
8. Aranki, A., S. A. Syed, E. B. Kenney, and R. Freter. 1969. Isolation of anaerobic bacteria from human gingiva and mouse secum by means of a simplified glove box procedure. Appl. Microbiol. 17:568–576.
9. Spaulding, E. H., V. Vargo, T. C. Michaelson, and R. M. Swenson. 1974. A comparison of two procedures for isolating anaerobic bacteria from clinical specimens. In A. Balows, R. M. Dehaan, V. R. Dowell, Jr., and L. B. Guze (eds.), Anaerobic Bacteria: Role in Disease, pp. 37–46. Charles C Thomas, Publisher, Springfield, Ill.
10. Rosenblatt, J. E., A. Fallon, and S. M. Finegold. 1973. Comparison of methods for isolation of anaerobic bacteria from clinical specimens. Appl. Microbiol. 25:77–85.
11. Starr, S. E. 1974. Comparison of Isolation Techniques for Anaerobic Bacteria. In A. Balows, R. M. Dehaan, V. R. Dowell, Jr., and L. B. Guze (eds.), Anaerobic Bacteria: Role in Disease, pp. 47–50. Charles C Thomas, Publisher, Springfield, Ill.
12. Gorbach, S. L., and J. G. Bartlett. 1974a. Anaerobic infections. New England J. Med. 290:1177–1184.
13. Gorbach, S. L., and J. G. Bartlett. 1974b. Anaerobic infections. New England J. Med. 290:1237–1245.
14. Gorbach, S. L., and J. G. Bartlett. 1974c. Anaerobic infections. New England J. Med. 290:1289–1294.
15. Gorbach, S. L., and J. G. Bartlett. 1974d. Anaerobic infections: Old myths and new realities. J. Infect. Dis. 130:307–310.
16. Martin, W. J. 1974. Isolation and identification of anaerobic bacteria in the clinical laboratory. A 2-year experience. Mayo Clin. Proc. 49:300–308.
17. Moore, W. E. C., E. P. Cato, and L. V. Holdeman. 1969. Anaerobic bacteria of the gastrointestinal flora and their occurrence in clinical infections. J. Infect. Dis. 119:641–649.
18. Sullivan, N. M., V. L. Sutter, M. M. Mims, V. H. Marsh, and S. M. Finegold. 1973. Clinical aspects of bacteremia after manipulation of the genitourinary tract. J. Infect. Dis. 127:49–55.
19. Washington, J. A., and W. J. Martin. 1973. Comparison of three blood culture media for recovery of anaerobic bacteria. Appl. Microbiol. 25:70–71.
20. Hobbs, G., K. Williams, and A. T. Willis. 1971. Basic methods for the isolation of clostridia. In D. A. Shapton and R. G. Board (eds.), The Society for Applied Bacteriology Technical Series No. 5, pp. 1–23. Academic Press, Inc., New York.

21. Martin, W. J. 1971. Practical method for isolation of anaerobic bacteria in the clinical laboratory. Appl. Mcrobiol. 22:1168–1171.

22. Ellner, P. D., P. A. Granato, and C. B. May. 1973. Recovery and identification of anaerobes: A system suitable for the routine clinical laboratory. Appl. Microbiol. 26:904–913.

23. Finegold, S. M., N. E. Harada, and L. G. Miller. 1967. Antibiotic susceptibility patterns as aids in classification and characterization of gram-negative anaerobic bacilli. J. Bact. 94:1443–1450.

24. Ninomiya, K., K. Suzuki, and S. Koosaka. 1970. Phenylethyl alcohol agar medium for isolation of anaerobic bacteria. Jap. J. M. S. & Biol. 23:403–411.

25. Sutter, V. L. and S. M. Finegold. 1971. Antibiotic disc susceptibility tests for rapid presumptive identification of gram-negative anaerobic bacilli. Appl. Microbiol. 21:13–20.

26. Moore, W. E. C., E. P. Cato and L. V. Holdeman. 1974. Identification of anaerobes from clinical infections. In A. Balows, R. M. Dehaan, V. R. Dowell, Jr., and L. B. Guze (eds.), Anaerobic Bacteria: Role in Disease, pp. 51–58. Charles C Thomas, Publisher, Springfield, Ill.

27. Starr, S. E., F. S. Thompson, V. R. Dowell, Jr., and A. Balows. 1973. Micromethod system for identification of anaerobic bacteria. Appl. Microbiol. 25:713–717.

28. Moore, H. G., V. L. Sutter, and S. M. Finegold. 1974. Comparison of three methods for biochemical testing of anaerobic bacteria. Presented at the 74th Annual Meeting of the American Society for Microbiology, May 12–17, Chicago, Ill.

29. Rahimi, A., W. J. Martin, and J. A. Washington II. 1974. Effects of medium and inoculum on antimicrobial susceptibility of anaerobic bacteria. Am. J. Clin. Path. 62:425–427.

30. Rosenblatt, J. E., and F. Schoenknecht. 1972. Effect of several components of anaerobic incubation on antibiotic susceptibility test results. Antimicrob. Agents Chemother. 1:433–440.

31. Sherris, J. C. 1974. A Discussion of Susceptibility Testing. In A. Balows, R. M. Dehaan, V. R. Dowell, Jr., and L. B. Guze (eds.), Anaerobic Bacteria: Role in Disease, pp. 497–503. Charles C Thomas, Publisher, Springfield, Ill.

32. Staneck, J. L., and J. A. Washington II. 1974. Antimicrobial susceptibilities of anaerobic bacteria: Recent clinical isolates. Antimicrob. Agents Chemother. 6:311–315.

33. Sutter, V. L., Y. Kwok, and S. M. Finegold. 1974. In Vitro Susceptibility Testing of Anaerobes: Standardization of a Single Disc Test. In A. Balows, R. M. Dehaan, V. R. Dowell, Jr., and L. B. Guze (eds.), Anaerobic Bacteria: Role in Disease, pp. 457–476. Charles C Thomas, Publisher, Springfield, Ill.

34. Thornsberry, C. 1974. Factors Affecting Susceptibility Tests and the Need for Standardized Procedures. In A. Balows, R. M. Dehaan, V. R. Dowell, Jr., and L. B. Guze (eds.), Anaerobic Bacteria: Role in Disease, pp. 477–486. Charles C Thomas, Publisher, Springfield, Ill.

35. Wilkins, T. D. 1974. Antibiotic Susceptibility Testing of Anaerobic Bacteria. In A. Balows, R. M. Dehaan, V. R. Dowell, Jr., and L. B. Guze (eds.), Anaerobic Bacteria: Role in Disease, pp. 451–455. Charles C Thomas, Publisher, Springfield, Ill.

36. Wilkins, T. D., L. V. Holdeman, I. J. Abramson, and W. E. C. Moore.

1972. Standardized single-disc method for antibiotic susceptibility testing of anaerobic bacteria. Antimicrob. Agents Chemother. 1:451–459.

37. Wilkins, T. D., and T. Thiel. 1973. Modified broth-disk method for testing the antibiotic susceptibility of anaerobic bacteria. Antimicrob. Agents Chemother. 3:350–356.

38. Martin, W. J., M. Gardner, and J. A. Washington II. 1972. In vitro antimicrobial susceptibility of anaerobic bacteria isolated from clinical specimens. Antimicrob. Agents Chemother. 1:148–158.

39. Stalons, D. R., C. Thornsberry, and A. Balows. 1974. Antimicrobial susceptibility testing of anaerobic bacteria. Presented at the 14th Interscience Conference on Antimicrobial Agents and Chemotherapy, September 11–13, San Francisco, Calif.

40. Sutter, V. L., Y. Kwok, and S. M. Finegold. 1973. Susceptibility of *Bacteroides fragilis* to six antibiotics determined by standardized antimicrobial disc susceptibility testing. Antimicrob. Agents Chemother. 3:188–193.

41. Fass, R. J., J. F. Scholand, G. R. Hodges, and S. Saslaw. 1973. Clindamycin in the treatment of serious anaerobic infections. Ann. Int. Med. 78:853–859.

42. Washington, J. A., W. J. Martin, and P. F. Hermans. 1974. In Vitro Susceptibility of Anaerobic Bacteria Isolated from Blood Cultures. *In* A. Balows, R. M. Dehaan, V. R. Dowell, Jr., and L. B. Guze (eds.), Anaerobic Bacteria: Role in Disease, pp. 487–496. Charles C Thomas, Publisher, Springfield, Ill.

43. Wilkins, T. D., and T. Thiel. 1973. Resistance of some species of *Clostridium* to clindamycin. Antimicrob. Agents Chemother. 3:136–137.

SECTION III

Systems for Clinical
Laboratory Immunology

Introduction

Chester M. Zmijewski

In preparing for this symposium, I realized that it has been 20 years since I was first introduced to the concept of clinical laboratory immunology in the serology laboratories of the Millard Fillmore Hospital in Buffalo, New York. In those days we were led to believe that such tests as the Weil-Felix reaction, slide tests for febrile agglutinins, heterophiles, and the highly complex Wasserman reaction were the quintessence of serological sophistication. As a matter of fact, some students spent a year or more trying to fathom the relationship of the colloidal gold test on spinal fluid to immunology, since this too was performed in the serology laboratory. Later, in bacteriology, we saw some equally awesome tests upon our first introduction to *Salmonella* and *Pneumococcus* typing. We were also made aware of the fact that some scientists at the university were capable of doing some equally mysterious tests on viruses in their clandestine laboratories.

Today, many of the old tests have been refined to increase their sensitivity and specificity to the point where they resemble only slightly the procedures which were held in such esteem. This revolution has been due, in large measure, to the rapid advancement of immunology. Many techniques now employed for routine clinical serological diagnosis had their beginnings in the research laboratories of investigators interested in basic immunobiological principles. Had it not been for the interest of a few astute individuals among them, who were able to see the ultimate value of some of these procedures as diagnostic tests, this symposium would be very boring indeed.

85

Fortunately, the work in the basic research laboratory on rabbits, guinea pigs, mice, and chickens did manage to filter down to the present day clinical laboratory. All of this happened in spite of several generations of vehemently protesting medical students who, at the time, could see no relationship whatsoever between such esoteric work and the diagnosis and treatment of sick people.

Now, we can see emerging a whole new breed of serology laboratories. These are capable of performing passive hemagglutination, immunoelectrophoresis, quantitative complement fixation, immunofluorescence, and radioimmunoassay, techniques that make the old ones look like child's play. This swing of the pendulum has been so great that there is a danger that the old methods might be completely forgotten. Certainly, we should not totally abandon the time-tested procedures since a portion of them have some usefulness because they are based on sound principles that are still valid. But newer methods must be introduced to make the job of serodiagnosis easier, faster, more accurate and meaningful, and in keeping with the wealth of our increasing knowledge of basic immunology.

This session can be considered as a kind of progress report to bring us up to date on several facets of serological testing. Dr. Palmer will discuss recent development in the serodiagnosis of mycotic infections, a group of diseases which have always presented problems to clinicians because of the time required for accurate laboratory diagnosis. Serodiagnostic tests for viral diseases will be presented by Dr. Plotkin and, hopefully, he will demonstrate that they are no longer mysterious and exclusively reserved for highly specialized research institutes. This is followed by Dr. Joncas' discussion on the laboratory diagnosis of infectious mononucleosis, and Dr. Rose will outline the latest details of tests for the diagnosis of autoimmune diseases.

CHAPTER 8

Immunological Diagnosis of Bacterial and Fungal Diseases

Dan F. Palmer

Development in the field of immunology over the past 12 years has resulted in significant progress in the techniques, instrumentation, and theory of serological tests. Furthermore, analysis of antibody responses in the light of expanded concepts concerning immunoglobulin structure and function has provided a more logical framework for interpreting serological data. Within the field of infectious disease serology, however, there has not been consistent acceptance of the newer techniques.

Currently, bacterial serology, with the exception of venereal disease (VD) serology, is a comparatively static field. Little change is being effected with regard to the serological procedures used in most laboratories for assaying antibodies to bacterial organisms. Fungal serology, on the other hand, has entered a period of considerable activity because new techniques are being used.

The distinction between the two fields is probably due, in large part, to contrasting levels of difficulty in isolating and identifying the respective infecting organisms. Because the etiological agent in bacterial disease can often be isolated and identified quickly and with a high rate of success, no urgent need for serodiagnostic criteria exists in most cases. In contrast, many mycotic infections are clinically indistinct, and isolation and identification of the infecting organism is time-consuming and difficult. Consequently, there is pressure to generate serological data to facilitate timely diagnoses of fungal diseases.

BACTERIAL SEROLOGY

The current status of bacterial serology is reflected in the list of procedures performed by clinical and public health laboratories for the assay of antibodies or other substances present in bacterial disease. These tests are shown in Table 1.

A. Enteric Bacteria

There are no new developments in the febrile agglutination tests. The Salmonella O and H agglutination tests continue to be condemned for nonspecificity and lack of standardization (1, 2), and emphasis is still placed on laboratory diagnosis by isolation and identification of the causative organism. Nevertheless, the majority of diagnostic laboratories still offer these tests for the clinician to develop presumptive data while awaiting isolation results. Some reference laboratories offer the agglutination test for Vi agglutinins for detecting and monitoring typhoid carriers. The validity of the test for detecting carriers is in doubt, however, because patients with typhoid fever may or may not develop Vi agglutinins.

B. Brucella and Fancisella

Agglutination tests for brucellosis and tularemia are given more credence than the others in the febrile series. Although a cross-agglutination relationship exists between *Brucella, Francisella,* and *Vibrio cholerae,* the tube or slide

Table 1. Current list of routine and reference serological tests for bacterial diseases (except syphilis)

1. "Febrile" agglutination tests
   Salmonella "O" agglutination
   Salmonella "H" agglutination
   Brucella agglutination
   Tularensis agglutination
2. Weil-Felix tests
   Proteus OX-19
   Proteus OX-2
   Proteus OX-K
3. Vi agglutination test
4. Streptococcal tests
   Antistreptolysin O
   Antihyaluronidase
   Antideoxyribonuclease B
5. Leptospira microscopic agglutination test
6. Listeria agglutination test
7. Tetanus and diphtheria hemagglutination tests

agglutination tests for brucellosis and tularemia yield useful information. Furthermore, standardization of the techniques is at least being attempted again, and there is a good standard antigen prepared by the National Animal Disease Laboratory and an international reference serum for brucella sero-diagnostic reagents.

Several commercial kits are available for detecting brucella antibodies by either the slide or tube tests, but most laboratories perform the slide test. A tabulation of recent proficiency test data obtained by the CDC (Table 2) indicates that, of 357 participating laboratories in the survey, 50% performed slide tests only, 24% performed tube tests only, and 26% performed both. Data from a similar program conducted by the College of American Patholo-gists (CAP) are shown in the same table; 84% of the laboratories participating in the CAP program performed slide tests, and only 12% performed tube tests. Tube tests for brucella antibodies yield, in general, 2-fold to 4-fold higher serum titers than do slide tests. This fact leads to the suspicion that tube tests would be better screening tests than slide tests, even though the latter were recommended for screening by the Committee on Public Health Aspects of Brucellosis, National Research Council, in 1954 (3). However, in at least one recent CDC proficiency test survey, the tube test resulted in more false negative reports on sera submitted to participating laboratories than did the slide test. This observation prompts a cautious approach to the question of which procedure is the most sensitive and specific.

The need to standardize procedure as well as reagents is obvious from the data in Table 3. In a survey taken in 1972, 100 laboratories participating in the CDC proficiency testing program reported varying conditions of incuba-tion in the brucella tube agglutination test. Some organizations conducting proficiency testing programs are currently contributing to the standardization of procedures when they report back to participating laboratories the meth-

Table 2. Brucella agglutination tests performed by laboratories participating in two proficiency testing programs

	CDC Program		CAP Program	
Test performed	No. of laboratories	%	No. of laboratories	%
Slide agglutination test	178	50	376	84
Tube agglutination test	85	24	55	12
Slide and tube test	94	26		
Not stated			15	3
Total laboratories	357		446	

Table 3. Conditions of incubation reported by 100 laboratories for Brucella tube test

No. of laboratories	Incubation temperature	Incubation duration (hr)
78	37°C	48
13	37°C	18–24
3	37°C	0.5
3	50–56°C	18–24
2	37°C	2
1	56°C	2

ods used by reference and referee laboratories. The participating laboratories tend to follow the lead of authorities in the field, and, thus, contribute to developing standards.

Serology for the assay of antibodies in tularemia is in a status similar to that of brucella serology, but there is no standard tularensis antigen. In contrast to brucella serology, tube and slide agglutination tests with tularensis antigen react to give approximately equal serum titers. The techniques used in tularensis agglutination tests also need to be standardized. The variations of incubation conditions existing in 102 laboratories surveyed in 1972 are illustrated in Table 4.

C. Rickettsia

The Weil-Felix tests are also in disrepute because they are nonspecific. The current recommendation in regard to these tests is to substitute the more specific rickettsial CF test in their place. Satisfactory rickettsial CF antigens are difficult to make and at present the market for them is not great. For these reasons, only a few companies are offering them for sale.

D. Streptococcus

For streptococcal serological testing, a new kit is now available to measure the serum level of antideoxyribonuclease B antibodies resulting from Group A streptococcal infection. Since the prevailing opinion among serologists is that at least two streptococcal serological tests should be performed to detect the highest number of streptococcal infections under practical circumstances, this new set of reagents is a welcome addition to the few tests available. The test involves the use of streptococcal enzyme deoxyribonuclease B and a substrate composed of highly polymerized deoxyribonucleic acid stained with methyl green. The action of the enzyme on its substrate is the depolymerization of the deoxyribonucleic acid (DNA), resulting in decolorization of the methyl green. A patient's serum added to the system prevents decolorization of the methyl green if antibodies against the enzyme are present. Normal

Table 4. Conditions of incubation reported by
102 laboratories for the tularensis tube agglutinat-
ing test

No. of laboratories	Incubation temperature	Incubation duration (hr)
38	37°C	24
42	37°C	2
	4−10°C	18
12	37°C	2
7	48−56°C	18
3	37°C	0.5

limits of antideoxyribonuclease B antibody titers are reported to be approximately the same as those for antistreptolysin O antibodies (4).

E. Leptospira

The leptospira microscopic agglutination test requires the laboratory to work
with live organisms, and, consequently, it is performed in reference laboratories only. A new indirect hemagglutination procedure is currently being
evaluated for leptospiral serology. The new procedure was developed as a
presumptive, or screening, test. It eliminates the need for live antigen, and a
few commercial companies have shown some interest in producing the reagents required for the test.

F. Listeria

Despite evidence that listeriosis is occurring with increasing frequency (5), the
listeria agglutination test is performed by very few reference laboratories in
this country. Interpretation of the test is complicated somewhat by the
existence of cross-reactions with *Staphylococcus aureus* antigen, and the sera
occasionally must be sorbed to remove the cross-reacting antibodies.

G. Syphilis

Tests for syphilis have undergone considerable evolution in the past decade.
The Venereal Disease Research Laboratory (VDRL) slide test is still the most
common screening and quantitating test for syphilis, but the rapid plasma
reagin (RPR) test is progressively replacing the VDRL test in laboratories for
these purposes. Table 5 lists the various tests performed by laboratories
participating in a proficiency testing program at CDC in September 1974.

Thirty-nine of the reporting laboratories used the automated reagin test
(ART) which employs the RPR card test antigen suspension in a continuous
flow AutoAnalyzer system. Tests are performed at the rate of 100/hr. The

Table 5. Syphilis serology tests performed by laboratories in the CDC proficiency testing program

Name of test	No. of laboratories performing
VDRL (qualitative and quantitative)	201
Rapid plasma reagin test (18 mm) (qualitative and quantitative)	113
Automated reagin test (qualitative and quantitative)	39
Unheated serum reagin test	14
FTA–ABS	132
Automated fluorescent treponemal antibody test	19
Microhemagglutination test for treponemal antibodies	5

trend in laboratories which receive large numbers of serum specimens for syphilis testing is in the direction of this automated system and the rapid reagin test.

Only 14 laboratories in the entire program are performing the unheated serum reagin test (USR), primarily because this test has no quantitative aspect. Furthermore, the USR test appears now to be slightly less sensitive than the VDRL test.

Of the specific treponemal antigen tests, the fluorescent treponemal antibody absorption test (FTA-ABS) is most extensively used at present. The test is used when questionable results are obtained with the preliminary tests, and although false-positive results can occur, it generally confirms the presence of treponemal antibodies. The test has been partially automated by using the SeroMatic System of Aerojet General Corporation,* and the automated test is comparable in specificity and sensitivity to the manual procedure. Slides processed automatically by the system must be examined manually, but the manufacturer states that as many as 200 tests/day can be performed. Nineteen of the 132 laboratories in Table 5 are currently using the automated procedure.

Finally, five laboratories reported using the new microhemagglutination test for Treponemal antibodies (MHA-TP) (6). In this test, tanned, formalinized sheep erythrocytes sensitized with treponemal antigen are used. The test has about the same specificity and sensitivity as the FTA-ABS test, except in early primary syphilis. There is some indication that the MHA-TP test is not as sensitive as the FTA-ABS in detecting early primary disease. This test can be automated by using automatic diluting instruments, such as the Autotiter equipment of Canalco, Inc. (7).

---

*Use of trade names is for identification only and does not constitute endorsement by the Public Health Service or by the U. S. Department of Health, Education, and Welfare.

In syphilis serology, the trend in cardiolipin tests is toward the simpler RPR and ART tests. The antigen used in these tests is stable. Practically everything needed to perform the RPR test is disposable, and these procedures are quite good for screening sera. In the confirmatory tests, the trend is toward the specific FTA-TP procedures. A commercial company is now marketing the MHA-TP confirmatory test in the form of a kit, and this may well increase the number of laboratories performing this procedure. It is still recommended that sera be screened with a cardiolipin test, such as the VDRL or RPR, followed by quantitation of sera exhibiting any degree of reactivity, and finally that diagnostic problem cases be tested with a confirmatory treponemal test, such as the FTA-ABS or MHA-TP.

H. Gonorrhea

No current serological tests for gonorrhea are suitable for routine screening of sera. Several tests have been developed in the past, but none has had adequate sensitivity or specificity. Therefore, the present recommendation is not to use serology as a substitute for established bacteriological culture techniques. Good serological tests are needed to detect gonococcal infections, and several groups are working on complement-fixation (CF) tests, indirect fluorescent antibody tests, radioimmunoassays, and other procedures in the hope of developing a more convenient screening method. Because of interest in the problem, perhaps not too much more time will elapse before an adequate serological method becomes available for detecting gonococcal antibody.

FUNGAL SEROLOGY

New techniques are being developed in fungal serology, and the CF, agglutination, and many precipitin tests now exist for many of the common mycoses. Numerous problems remain to be solved in this area of practical serology, however, and extensive studies are still needed for practical, unequivocal tests. Furthermore, commercial sources of diagnostic reagents are needed for several of the tests already in use.

Table 6 lists the serological tests currently used for eight of the more common mycoses. Note that immunodiffusion is now used quite extensively. Not long ago immunodiffusion was limited in most laboratories to use as an adjunct to the CF test for the serodiagnosis of histoplasmosis. Immunodiffusion tests have also been developed for aspergillosis, blastomycosis, candidiasis, coccidioidomycosis, and paracoccidioidomycosis.

The CF test is still used as an aid in diagnosing all of the diseases listed except candidiasis and sporotrichosis, but insensitive and nonspecific reactions are often involved with this test. Other methods listed are tube precipi-

Table 6. List of serological tests and commercial availability of reagents

Disease	Serological tests used	Commercial reagent availability
Aspergillosis	Immunodiffusion CF	None MBA[a]
Blastomycosis	Immunodiffusion CF	None MBA
Candidiasis	Immunodiffusion Agglutination Latex agglutination	A skin test antigen from Hollister-Stier can be used A skin test antigen from Hollister-Stier can be used
Coccidioidomycosis	Immunodiffusion CF Latex agglutination Tube precipitin test	Hyland Kit MBA, Microbiological Consulting Service Hyland Kit Heated CF antigen can be used
Cryptococcosis	CF Charcoal agglutination Agglutination Latex agglutination IFA	None None None Kit from Industrial Biological Laboratories None
Histoplasmosis	Immunodiffusion CF (Mycelial and yeast) Latex agglutination	Concentrated CF antigen can be used MBA Kit from Colab, Hyland
Paracoccidioidomycosis	Immunodiffusion CF Tube precipitin test	None None None
Sporotrichosis	Tube agglutination Latex agglutination	None None

[a]Microbiological Associates.

tin, latex or charcoal agglutination, agglutination, and indirect fluorescent antibody.

A. Commercial Reagents

The column in Table 6 indicating commercial availability of the test reagents reflects a growing interest by some companies in producing these reagents. Although no reagents are yet available for paracoccidioidomycosis and sporotrichosis, some are on the market for performing one or more tests for the other diseases listed. Very recently, a fungal reagent test kit was marketed by Microbiological Associates to aid in the serodiagnosis of histoplasmosis, blastomycosis, coccidioidomycosis, and aspergillosis. This kit contains antigens for use in the CF test, hemolysin, complement, and microtitration plates. Both mycelial and yeast phase histoplasma antigens are included. Microbiological Consulting Service, Long Beach, California, also has marketed a CF antigen for coccidioidomycosis.

Hyland Laboratories of Costa Mesa, California market latex agglutination kits for coccidioidomycosis and histoplasmosis, and an immunodiffusion kit for coccidioidomycosis. A latex agglutination kit for cryptococcosis is available from Industrial Biological Laboratories, Rockville, Maryland, and Consolidated Laboratories, Glenwood, Illinois, in addition to Hyland, produces a latex agglutination kit for histoplasmosis.

Finally, Hollister-Stier Laboratories of Spokane, Washington, market a skin test antigen for candidiasis which can be used to sensitize latex particles for the latex agglutination test and also can be used in an immunodiffusion test for detecting Candida antibodies.

Considering the current aspects of serodiagnosis for individual mycoses, it becomes evident that even though a number of tests are available to detect antibodies in each disease, results are often merely presumptive and, because of low sensitivity, negative results do not rule out a positive diagnosis.

B. Aspergillosis

The double diffusion test may be used for the serodiagnosis of some forms of the disease, but not for others. Antibodies can be demonstrated in almost all patients with aspergillomas, in approximately 70% of patients with the allergic form of the disease, and in a few patients with invasive aspergillosis. The CF test is less specific than the immunodiffusion test, but it has been found to be useful in detecting active or very recent infection. In general, serodiagnosis of aspergillosis is based principally on the immunodiffusion technique because of its high specificity. Unfortunately, the technique is not sensitive enough. Studies are being conducted on the use of counterelectrophoresis to provide more rapid and possibly more sensitive results. Furthermore, the indirect fluorescent antibody test is being examined for possible use in this disease.

C. Blastomycosis

The CF test for this disease lacks sufficient specificity, reacts frequently with sera from patients with coccidioidomycosis and histoplasmosis, and also lacks sensitivity in that less than half of the sera from patients with blastomycosis react in the test. On the other hand, the immunodiffusion test permits a more specific diagnosis of blastomycosis in approximately 80% of patients with the disease (8) when reference sera containing both A and B precipitins are used as controls.

D. Candidiasis

Immunodiffusion, agglutination, and latex agglutination are used for the diagnosis of systemic candidiasis. Immunodiffusion with the somatic antigen is now the most widely accepted technique, although the latex agglutination test has greater sensitivity. Unfortunately, the latex agglutination test also reacts for some patients with cryptococcosis and tuberculosis (9). The yeast cell agglutination test is also useful for detecting active candidiasis when changing titers in serial specimens can be demonstrated. Some experimental work on indirect hemagglutination and immunofluorescence is being conducted currently.

E. Coccidioidomycosis

The serological tests indicated for coccidioidomycosis have proved quite valuable for detecting and monitoring cases of this disease. The tube precipitin test is most valuable for detecting early primary disease or exacerbated existing disease, but the CF test detects a number of infections missed by the tube precipitin test. The immunodiffusion and latex agglutination tests are considered screening tests with fair sensitivity, but they occasionally yield false positive results.

F. Paracoccidioidomycosis

CF and immunodiffusion tests are currently the most widely accepted procedures for paracoccidioidomycosis. When these two tests are used concurrently, over 95% of the cases of this disease can be detected serologically (11).

G. Cryptococcosis

This disease usually is diagnosed serologically by detecting polysaccharide capsular antigen in body fluids by the latex agglutination test. This test is specific, highly sensitive, and prognostic. When antigen is absent or present in small amounts antibody may be detected by any of the other tests listed. Maximal serological diagnosis of cryptococcosis is reported to be accomplished by employing three tests: the latex agglutination test for cryptococcal antigen, and the indirect fluorescent antibody and tube agglutination tests for antibodies (10).

H. Histoplasmosis

Current practice for achieving serodiagnostic coverage in histoplasmosis is CF with both mycelial and yeast phase antigens, supplemented by the immunodiffusion test. The latex agglutination test, commercially available in the form of a kit, is not considered a replacement for the CF test but may be used with anticomplementary sera.

I. Sporotrichosis

Finally, the tube agglutination and latex agglutination tests are now known to be useful for the serodiagnosis of various forms of sporotrichosis. Both tests are reliable, but the latex agglutination test appears to be more sensitive and specific. Best diagnostic coverage is probably achieved by the combined use of both tests (12).

The trend in fungal serology appears to be directed toward developing serological methods which can resolve specific and nonspecific reactions. Thus, the immunodiffusion tests can, in many cases, provide the analytical power required to identify specific antigen-antibody systems, and the fungal serologists are taking advantage of this characteristic to alleviate some of the problems caused by cross-reacting antigens among the pathogenic fungi.

LITERATURE CITED

1. Schroder, S. A. 1968. Interpretation of serologic tests for typhoid fever. J.A.M.A. 206:839–840.
2. Reynolds, D. W., R. L. Carpenter, and W. H. Simon. 1970. Diagnostic specificity of Widal's reaction for typhoid fever. J.A.M.A. 214:2192–2193.
3. Spink, W. W., N. B. McCullough, L. M. Hutchings, and C. K. Mingle. 1954. A standardized antigen and agglutination technique for human brucellosis. Am. J. Clin. Path. 24:496–498.
4. Klein, G., C. Baker, and W. Jones. 1971. Upper limits of normal antistreptolysin O and antideoxyribonuclease B titers. Appl. Microbiol. 21:999–1001.
5. Busch, L. A. 1971. Human listeriosis in the United States 1967–1969. J. Infect. Dis. 123:328–332.
6. Logan, L. C., and P. M. Cox. 1970. Evaluation of a quantitative automated microhemagglutination assay for antibodies to *Treponema pallidum*. Am. J. Clin. Pathol. 53:163.

7. Coffee, E. M., L. L. Bradford, L. S. Naritomi, and R. M. Wood. 1972. Evaluation of the qualitative and automated quantitative microhemaggluti-nation assay for antibodies to *Treponema pallidum.* Appl. Microbiol. 24:26.
8. Kaufman, L., D. W. McLaughlin, M. J. Clark, and S. Blumer. 1973. Specific immunodiffusion test for blastomycosis. Appl. Microbiol. 26:244–247.
9. Kaufman, L. 1974. Serodiagnosis of fungal diseases. *In* E. H. Lennette, E. H. Spaulding, and J. P. Truant (eds.), Manual of Clinical Microbiology, Ed. 2, pp. 557–568. American Society for Microbiology, Washington, D.C.
10. Kaufman, L., and S. Blumer. 1968. Value and interpretation of serological tests for the diagnosis of cryptococcosis. Appl. Microbiol. 16:1907–1912.
11. Restrepo, M. A., and L. H. Moncada F. 1970. Serologic procedures in the diagnosis of paracoccidioidomycosis. Proceedings of the International Symposium on Mycoses. Scientific Publication of the Pan-American Health Organization. No. 205, pp. 101–110.
12. Karlin, J. V., and H. S. Nielsen. 1970. Serologic aspects of sporotricho-sis. J. Infect. Dis. 121:316–327.

CHAPTER 9

Rapid Diagnosis of Viral Infections

Stanley A. Plotkin

Since diagnostic virology is not undertaken by most clinical microbiology laboratories, the subject for them remains somewhat arcane. Nevertheless, diagnostic virology is beginning to develop into a significant clinical laboratory subject. In the past, it has been justifiably considered a specialized, academic procedure of little relevance to the treatment of patients. Now, however, specific diagnosis of some viral infections has value for selection of therapy and it is urgent that a methodology be devised to give clinicians answers as rapidly as possible. Hospitals with comprehensive clinical laboratories, therefore, should have diagnostic virology facilities and it is feasible, in many cases, to incorporate them into existing microbiology laboratories.

Since it is impossible to cover the entire field of diagnostic virology, I would like to stress the diagnosis of those diseases that lend themselves to intervention, or at least the diagnosis of which leads to certain prognostic implications. Unfortunately, in virology, there is no such thing as that invaluable medium of the bacteriologist, blood agar: in other words, no medium that will support the growth of most viruses. Therefore, multiple techniques are needed for virus isolation. Fortunately, however, it is generally agreed that most of the common human pathogenic viruses can be isolated by using three types of cell culture: first, primary cultures of kidney cells from monkeys, such as rhesus or African green; second, culture of a continuous cell line of strains of human fibroblasts such as WI-38; and third, a continuous cell line of the Hela cell variety (many laboratories prefer HEP-2). With these three types of cell cultures, and the occasional use of suckling mice, one can isolate most of the important human viral pathogens.

After isolation, the task of identification is best handled by sending the isolate to reference laboratories such as those operated by state public health departments. If state laboratories were sent only positive isolates, their facilities would be more productively utilized. It is impractical for any state laboratory to receive poorly collected, poorly verified heterogenous collections of specimens and then to test them by expensive procedures with an expectation of a yield of only 3% or less.

If more hospitals had virus-isolation facilities, a presumptive diagnosis could be returned to the clinicians promptly. Such presumptive diagnoses can frequently be made simply from the type of cytopathogenic effect (CPE) that the viruses exhibit in tissue cultures (1). For example, some viruses, such as cytomegalovirus (CMV), have a very characteristic CPE in cultures of WI-38; when these specific foci are seen, a reasonably accurate diagnosis can be made; the presence of adenovirus is revealed by a grape-like rounding of the cells in all three types of tissue cultures mentioned; and herpesvirus is easily recognized by its rapid growth and complete CPE in human as well as other cell cultures. There are some myxoviruses that do not cause CPE, but can be detected by the simple phenomenon of hemadsorption. Myxoviruses such as parainfluenza change the surface of the cell so that they adsorb to the surface of the tissue culture medium. The technique simply is to place a suspension of red cells on the infected cell cultures, to incubate the cultures, to wash after incubation, and to look for hemadsorbing agents that can then be specifically identified by neutralization. The point is that, with a few cell lines and a conscientious trained technician, viruses can be isolated even in laboratories that are not primarily virus diagnostic laboratories.

A more specific problem, and one which I have to deal with constantly at Children's Hospital, is that of the diagnosis of congenital infections, labeled "the TORCH syndrome," and including toxoplasmosis, rubella, CMV, and herpes. In terms of the incidence of these diseases, I really think the acronym should have been "crotch," since CMV virus is by far the most important, rubella being second, and with toxoplasmosis, coxsackie B, and herpes occurring in descending order.

VIRAL DIAGNOSTIC PROCEDURES

A. Cytomegalovirus

The diagnosis of CMV virus infection has become very important because of the epidemiological finding that 1% of all infants are born infected with CMV; that is, they have sustained an intrauterine infection. Of this 1%, it appears that no less than 10% suffer mental retardation as the result of this infection. Statistics on permanent damage may turn out eventually to be even higher, especially when some degree of hearing loss is included in the total assessment of damage. Both virus isolation procedures and serological procedures are available to diagnose CMV in the newborn. The virus isolation procedure depends upon the use of cell strains of human fibroblasts which are commercially available in tubes or flasks. These cells are inoculated with urine from the newborn. Since congenitally infected infants almost uniformly excrete large amounts of virus, it is usually not necessary to incubate the cultures for weeks or months, and positive results can be had 3 or 4 days after inoculation.

In addition, there are a few serological tests which are widely used for the diagnosis of CMV. One is the complement fixation test which depends on the availability of the virus strain AD-169, a strain that has a broad antigenic reactivity and will react with 90% of sera from infants born with congenital CMV infection. Since the infants have usually been infected for 6 to 8 months in utero, there will be high complement fixing antibody titers at birth, perhaps in the range of 1:64 or greater. The mother, of course, will also have a high titer.

The most specific test for immunity to CMV infection is the indirect immunofluorescence test. For this test, one obviously has to have a fluorescent microscope and a technician familiar with its operation and with the pitfalls of the test. Briefly, the test for indirect fluorescent antibodies against CMV involves fixing CMV-infected cells on slides, placing the patient's serum over the cells, followed by a fluorescent antihuman globulin. There is a kit available commercially but, unfortunately, in my experience, it has given very poor results and I cannot recommend it. It is not difficult, however, to make up slides bearing CMV-infected cells using the multiple chambers known by the name of Lab-Tek. There are two important technical points. One is the use of a detergent such as NP40 to open the cells to staining and the other is the use of Evans blue as a counterstain. With the right fluorescent antiglobulins, one can look for total CMV antibodies, IgG CMV antibodies, or IgM CMV antibodies. The identification of IgM antibody assures one that the antibody detected in the infant is the result of infection and is not passive antibody. On the other hand, there are cases where IgM antibodies are not detected and where follow-up titers and virus isolation must precede diagnosis.

The diagnosis of a congenital infection with herpesvirus depends on virus isolation and not on serology. Since herpesvirus grows rapidly and in many cell lines, its isolation should pose no real difficulty.

B. Rubella

The test for rubella antibodies is probably the most widely used viral serology procedure in this country. Although this technique has been very successful in identifying seronegatives, there are pitfalls to avoid, particularly in failure to remove inhibitors. I would not particularly recommend one kit over another, although we use 1-day-old chick cells in preference to tannic acid-treated human cells. The fixed chick cells sold by Abbott seem to compare favorably with fresh chick cells. We prefer to use heparin-$MnCl_2$ to remove inhibitors rather than kaolin. One of the most important things to remember about rubella serology is that any laboratory doing the test should be prepared to keep sera for at least 6 months to be retested with a second specimen if the necessity should arise.

C. Toxoplasmosis

For antibodies to the protozoan, toxoplasmosis, a kit from the Electro-nucleonics Company has given us very satisfactory results in identifying total antibodies by indirect fluorescence. Fortunately, in toxoplasmosis, one can make a presumptive diagnosis with one serum because only 1% of asymptomatic individuals will have titers comparable to those of congenitally infected individuals. For positive diagnosis it may be desirable, in addition, to have an IgM toxoplasmosis antibody test done by a reference laboratory such as the Bureau of Laboratories of the CDC.

D. Respiratory Viruses

The fact that most respiratory infections are of viral etiology is well known. Nevertheless, many of these infections are futilely treated with antibiotics because a positive diagnosis of viral infection cannot be made with sufficient rapidity. As commercial reagents become available, the use of indirect fluorescence should soon remedy that deficiency. It will then become possible to identify the most ubiquitous viral pathogens of childhood, which are the respiratory syncytial virus (RSV) (which causes bronchiolitis), parainfluenza viruses (which cause croup), adenoviruses, and influenza viruses. Specimens can be collected according to the following method developed by Garner (2). A polyethylene tube small enough to pass the infant's nostril is passed into the nasopharynx, and mucus is aspirated by vacuum into a collector. This material is kept cold and mixed with enough saline solution to dilute the mucus. The cells are sedimented by centrifugation, the supernatant is discarded, and the cells are resuspended in saline to produce a suspension containing sufficient cells to make slides. The slides are then dried and finally fixed with cold acetone. Direct fluorescent antibodies are used to identify virus antigen in the cells using reagents consisting of guinea pig antisera to the important viruses.

A study of bronchiolitis in England (2) compared the use of FA testing to identify a virus with the use of standard virus isolation techniques. Of 75 cases studied, RSV was isolated from the nasopharynx in 74 cases; RSV-antigen was identified by FA test in 71 cases; and 1 case was FA-positive, in which virus was not isolated. The accuracy of the FA technique is, therefore, demonstrably high.

To make FA testing more practical, intersecting pools of antisera can be prepared combining influenza A and B, parainfluenza type 1, *Herpes simplex*, RSV, mumps, adenoviruses, and *Mycoplasma pneumonia* in various ways. By this means, one can presumptively identify the antigen present in the respiratory secretion. A report from Baylor University compared indirect fluorescence testing with tissue culture isolation: of a total of 52 specimens, 45 cases were positive both in tissue culture and by indirect fluorescence and identified influenza, parainfluenza, RSV adenovirus, and herpesviruses. In four cases, tissue culture was not successful in isolating virus although FA was positive. In three cases (all adenoviruses), FA was negative but tissue culture was positive. Thus, a majority of viral respiratory infections can be identified using the FA technique and this could save thousands of dollars now being spent on useless antibiotic treatment of viral infection, especially in infants.

E. Hepatitis

With regard to the diagnosis of hepatitis, the detection of hepatitis B antigen in blood banks is routine and involves radioimmunoassay (RIA) or reverse passive hemagglutination techniques, both of which utilize commercially available kits. The reverse passive hemagglutination is a particularly simple technique and is almost as accurate as RIA.

Certain other tests are probably required to detect chronic carriers of hepatitis B since the hepatitis B particle is composed of two antigens: the core antigen and the surface antigen. The surface antigen is in tremendous excess in serum and is detected by the usual tests for hepatitis B antigen. However, epidemiological studies show clearly that most units of blood capable of transmitting hepatitis B do not have detectable antigen, even in RIA. With the most sensitive methods for detection of antigen, only 30–50% of donor blood units carrying hepatitis B viruses are identified. Another test may identify those chronic carriers of hepatitis B who do not have detectable levels of surface antigen in their serum—a test to demonstrate antibody to the core material of the virus. All virus carriers have circulating core antibodies (3). The core antigen can be derived from complete virus (Dane) particles present in blood or infected liver. Anticore antibodies have been detected by complement fixation, radioimmunoprecipitation, and by fluorescence on sections of infected liver. A patient with acute hepatitis B will develop core antibodies early in infection, but this core antibody will decline at the time antibody to the surface antigen appears. If, on the other hand, the patient develops into a chronic carrier, he will continue to have core antibody and will not develop antibody to the surface antigen. Therefore, the core antibody technique can detect chronic carriers whether or not they have positive tests for antigen. Such detection is badly needed and one hopes that the new reagents will become commercially available.

F. Encephalitides

The last points I will make concern the diagnosis of the chronic encephalitides, subacute sclerosing panencephalitis (SSPE) and herpes encephalitis, caused by the measles virus and *Herpes simplex* respectively. Both of these can be diagnosed by isolation of virus from the brain, but isolation takes time. In the case of SSPE, the diagnosis can be made by demonstration of high serum or CSF antibody to measles, but a rapid diagnosis can be obtained by taking cells from the spinal fluid, centrifuging them, and applying the indirect FA technique to detect measles antigen in the cells (4). In possible herpes virus infection, the staining of cells from the spinal fluid or, when a brain biopsy is done, indirect fluorescence on a section of the brain, are much more rapid and specific diagnostic techniques than even virus isolation, because, in some cases, although viral antigens are present, infectious virus may be absent (5).

LITERATURE CITED

1. Walker, W. E., R. R. Martins, P. A. Karrels, and R. W. Gay. 1971. Rapid clinical diagnosis of common viruses by specific cytopathic changes in unstained tissue culture roller tubes. Am. J. Clin. Path. 56:384–393.
2. Sturdy, P. M., J. McQuillin, and P. S. Gardner. 1969. A comparative study of methods for the diagnosis of respiratory virus infections in childhood. J. Hyg. 67:659.
3. Hoofnagle, J. H., R. J. Gerety, and L. F. Barker. 1973. Antibody to hepatitis B virus core in man. Lancet 2:869–873.
4. Dayan, A. D., and M. I. Stokes. 1971. Immunofluorescent detection of measles-virus antigens in cerebrospinal-fluid cells in subacute sclerosing panencephalitis. Lancet 1:891–892.
5. Liu, C., and R. Llanes-Rodas. 1972. Application of the immunofluorescent technique to the study of pathogenesis and rapid diagnosis of viral infections. Am. J. Clin. Path. 57:829–834.

CHAPTER 10

Laboratory Diagnosis of Infectious Mononucleosis: Epstein–Barr Virus and the Heterophil Test

Jean H. Joncas*

The diagnosis of infectious mononucleosis rests upon the detection of characteristic heterophil agglutinins in the serum of patients with the disease (1, 2). In the past few years, slide tests using horse red cells have been devised in an attempt to make the diagnosis of infectious mononucleosis easier and faster (3, 4). The use of horse red cells instead of sheep red cells in tube tests or in microtiter tests was recently recommended since the test using horse cells, providing differential absorption is carried out, is more sensitive and just as reliable (4). Finally, the Epstein-Barr virus-viral capsid antigen (EBV-VCA antibodies) detected by indirect immunofluorescence were found to be present in virtually all cases of heterophil positive infectious mononucleosis, as well as in a certain number of heterophil negative cases of the disease (5–8). The Epstein-Barr virus-early antigen diffuse type (EBV-EA-D antibodies) and the EBV-IgM antibodies may also be useful in the diagnosis of infectious mononucleosis, but there is comparatively little data on the prevalence of these antibodies to date (9–14). Recently, the combination of a positive VCA antibody test with a negative Epstein-Barr nuclear antigen (EBNA) antibody test early in the course of infectious mononucleosis has been found useful in the diagnosis of this disease (15). The present work was undertaken to compare the relative value of each of these tests in the diagnosis of infectious mononucleosis and to determine the lifespan of these various antibodies.

---

*Work reported performed with F. Gervais, M. Leyritz, and R. Robitaille.

METHODS

The following material was available for the study: 244 sera from 108 cases of infectious mononucleosis, 93 of which were heterophil positive using sheep cells and 15 of which were heterophil negative by the same test. An additional number of 304 sera from 280 cases admitted to hospital or seen in the outpatient department with a variety of infectious and noninfectious syndromes were submitted to the same test.

Sheep cell and horse cell heterophil agglutinins were measured by the Paul Bunnell Davidsohn test in microtiter plates (1, 4). The microtiter plates used and the results obtained in a typical case of mononucleosis are shown in Figure 1. The first three horizontal rows of wells have been used for the test with sheep red blood cells without prior absorption of the serum (*first row*), following beef red cell absorption (*second row*), and following guinea pig kidney absorption (*third row*). The fourth and fifth horizontal rows, rows D and E, have been used for the determination of horse red cell agglutinins following beef red cell absorption and guinea pig kidney absorption respectively. The criteria used for positivity were those of Davidsohn and Lee (1). The sheep cell agglutinin titer should be at least 1:28 prior to absorption, providing it was still at least 1:7 following guinea pig kidney absorption and negative at the 1:7 dilution following beef red cell absorption. When the presumptive titer was higher than 1:28, this titer did not fall more than three tube dilutions following guinea pig kidney absorption and did fall at least four tube dilutions or more following beef red cell absorption. The test with horse cells is considered positive if the titer following guinea pig kidney absorption is at least one dilution higher than following beef red cell absorption.

Two slide tests were also used for the determination of horse cell agglutinins, the monospot and the monotest. The monospot kit contains a guinea pig kidney reagent, a beef red cell reagent, and a positive control serum, but no negative control serum. Stabilized horse red blood cells are used as indicator cells. The test should be read within 60 sec and a positive serum should show an agglutination following absorption with the first reagent but no agglutination following absorption with a second reagent. Any other results are considered negative.

The monotest kit contains a positive and a negative control serum in addition to stabilized horse red blood cells as indicator cells. Agglutination should occur with these cells if the serum tested gives a titer of 1:56 or greater in the standard Paul Bunnell presumptive test using sheep red blood cells without prior differential absorption. Agglutination with the unknown serum tested in the center of the slide is compared with the agglutination obtained on the same slide on the left with the positive control serum and on the right with the negative control serum. The test should be read within 2 min.

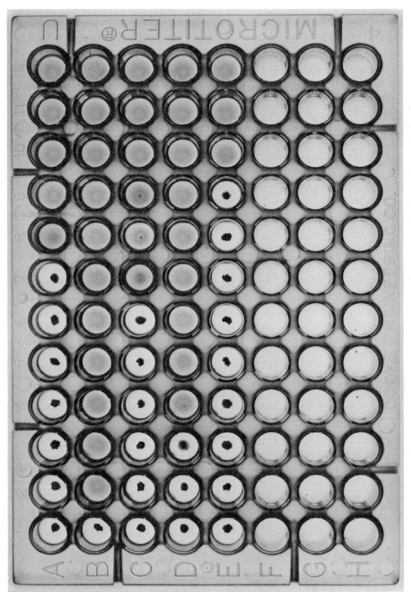

Figure 1. Microtiter plates used and results obtained in a typical case of mononucleosis.

The EBV-VCA and EA antibodies were measured by indirect immuno-fluorescence (14). The EBV-VCA antibody titers were measured by indirect immunofluorescence in 2-fold dilutions from 1:5 to 1:320 with the use of the HRIK clone of P3J lymphoblastoid cells as antigen positive cells and Hyland fluorescein-conjugated goat antiserum to human IgG (heavy and light chain specific). Raji lymphoblastoid cells were used as antigen negative control cells. Known positive and negative sera were used as control sera.

The EBV-EA antibody titers were measured by a similar indirect immuno-fluorescence test on acetone-fixed Raji cells, 5 days following bromodeoxy-uridine (BUdR) induction of the EBV-EA antigens. Control tests included a VCA positive, EA negative serum on BUdR-activated Raji cells and a VCA positive, EA positive serum on normal antigen negative RAji cells and on BUdR-activated Raji cells. The EBNA antibody titers were measured follow-ing the modification suggested by Henle, Henle, and Horwitz (15) of a method originally described by Reedman and Klein (16).

Specific EBV-IgM antibodies were measured on acetone-fixed HRIK lym-phoblastoid cells by a modification of a method described by Schmitz and Scherer (12), on unfractionated whole serum as well as on the corresponding IgM fraction following sucrose density gradient centrifugation. Twelve frac-tions of approximately 0.3 ml each were collected from the gradient, and their IgM and IgG contents were determined by radial immunodiffusion using Behringwerke (Hoesch Pharmaceutical) or Hyland immunoplates. Fractions shown to contain only IgM or only IgG by this method were pooled and tested in parallel with the corresponding whole serum for EB virus-specific IgM and IgG antibodies by the indirect immunofluorescence techniques. The dilution resulting from the sucrose density gradient separation was found to approximate 1:5. Sera were absorbed on boiled beef red cells before the test. IgM fractions from known IgM positive and IgM negative sera and correspond-ing IgG fractions were used as controls. Hyland unconjugated goat antihuman IgM (μ chain specific) antiserum and fluorescein-conjugated rabbit antigoat 7S gamma globulin antiserum were used as second and third coat in this three-coat sandwich technique as described by Schmitz and Scherer (12). In a preliminary experiment (Table 1), 1 ml of a 1:16 dilution of the goat antihuman IgM reagent was mixed with variable amounts (0.01 mg–6 mg) of Cohn fraction II (Nutritional Biochemical Co., lot no. 6945) for 1 hr at 37°C and overnight at 4°C. It was, subsequently, centrifuged at 2500 g for 30 min. The supernatant was collected and the sediment was discarded. This step in the procedure was found to be the single most important factor in arriving at specific reproducible results in the IgM test. In addition, each lot of anti-human IgM antiserum was screened for blocking activity on the IgM produc-ing Daudi or Dubois lymphoblastoid cell lines stained by Hyland fluorescein-conjugated goat antihuman immunoglobulin (heavy and light chain specific) antiserum. Antihuman IgM antisera unable to block at the 1:5 dilution in this screening test were not found satisfactory for the IgM antibody test. In rare

Table 1. Effect of absorption of the goat antihuman IgM reagent with Cohn Fraction II on the EBV-IgM specific antibody titer and nonspecific fluorescence

	Amount of Cohn fraction (mg)							EBV-VCA (IgG) antibody titer[a]
	0.00	0.01	0.1	0.5	1	3	6	
Cells								
1. Sera or fractions								
2. Goat antihuman IgM								
3. Rabbit antigoat globulin conjugate								
HRIK antigen positive cells								
Control IgG fraction (J.B.) (+2 +3)	>10	>10	5	Neg.	Neg.	Neg.	Neg.	320
Negative control serum (J.J.) (+2 +3)	>10	>10	Neg.	Neg.	Neg.	Neg.	Neg.	40
Positive control serum (I.B.) (+2 +3)	80	80	40	20	10	10	10	320
Positive control[b] IgM fraction (J.B.) (+2 +3)	80	40	40	10	20	10	10	80

[a]EBV-VCA, Epstein-Barr virus-viral capsid antigen. The EBV-VCA antibody titer was measured by indirect immunofluorescence using Hyland goat anti-IgG (heavy and light chain specific) conjugate.
[b]When the Cohn fraction II-absorbed anti-IgM reagent was also absorbed by the same procedure on the positive control IgM fraction (J.B.), the anti-IgM reagent could no longer give any fluorescence on EBV-IgM positive control serum or fractions.

instances where the EBV-VCA IgG antibody titer exceeds 1:1,000, it is preferable to do the IgM test on the IgM fraction rather than on the unfractionated serum or to remove the excess IgG from the serum to be tested by a method recently described by Ankerst et al. (17).

RESULTS

The horse cell agglutinin microtiter test appeared to be more sensitive than the sheep cell agglutinin test since all cases of infectious mononucleosis, whether heterophil positive or negative by sheep cells, were positive by horse cells (Table 2). The specificity of the horse cell agglutinin test was extremely good since only 2% of 280 controls were shown to have a detectable titer of these agglutinins. In at least 3 of the 15 heterophil negative cases (cases A. L. S., C. B., and B. G., Table 3) from which sera were still available, the detection of specific EBV-IgM antibodies strongly suggested a diagnosis of infectious mononucleosis. Furthermore, in at least three of the controls, positive for these horse cell agglutinins (for example, cases S. B., and M. M.), the detection of either IgM antibodies or EA antibodies strongly suggested asymptomatic recent EBV infection. In view of the very high sensitivity of the horse cell agglutinin test and its relatively long lifespan, as shown in Figure 2, it is even surprising that so few positive tests were encountered among the controls. Indeed, horse red cells gave titers on the average of two dilutions higher than sheep red cells. Furthermore, in two cases of infectious mononucleosis, horse cell agglutinins appeared earlier than sheep cell agglutinins and, in several cases, persisted for much longer periods than sheep cell agglutinins, as long as 21 and 23 months in two cases. The interpretation, therefore, of a positive test either on slide or in microtiter tests using horse erythrocytes, is difficult. Such a positive test may result from the persistence of agglutinins detectable by this sensitive test following a clinically apparent or inapparent mononucleosis months before. In rare cases, it may represent a true false positive test as it was, presumably, in the two cases positive by monotest in Table 4. These two positive tests were encountered in a case of varicella and in a case of influenza A Hong Kong virus infection. On the other hand, false negative monotests were encountered in 12 cases. In 10 of these 12 cases, however, the sheep cell agglutinin titer in microtiter tests was low, being 28 before absorption, staying at the same titer or at a titer superior to 1:7 following guinea pig kidney absorption, but becoming undetectable following beef red cell absorption (case N. R., Table 3). In the other two, the unabsorbed titers were 56 and 112 respectively. These low positive titers apparently cannot be detected by the monotest, except possibly if the slide is examined under the microscope as we have done in several of these cases (Table 5). In three of these cases, in which the EBV-IgM antibody test was

Table 2. Horse red blood cell agglutinins in microtiter tests in cases of infectious mononucleosis and in controls

Cases and sera	Horse cell agglutinins (microtiter test) No. of sera with an absorbed titer (GPK)[a]			Positive cases (%)
	<7 or negative	<56	>56	
108 cases of mononucleosis with 244 sera				
93 cases with 169 het. pos.[b] sera	0[c]	14 (12)[d]	155 (49)	100
with 56 het. neg.[b] sera (in follow-up)	0	41 (19)	15 (15)	
15 cases with 19 het. neg. sera	0	6 (6)	13 (9)	100
280 controls with 304 sera (all het. neg.)	295 (272)	6 (6)	2 (2)	2

[a]GPK, titer following absorption on guinea pig kidney in cases where it was higher than after absorption on boiled beef red cells (BBRC). If found higher after BBRC than after GPK, the test was read as negative.

[b]Het. pos., heterophil positive; het. neg., heterophil negative. By Standard Paul Bunnell Davidsohn test with sheep cells.

[c]0, none found; all sera tested.

[d]( ), no. of cases.

Table 3. Comparison of nonspecific heterophil agglutinins and specific EBV antibodies in selected cases

Cases	Age (yr)	Days after onset of disease	Group	Sheep cell agglutinin titer			Horse cell agglutinin titer		MT[e]	MS[f]	EBV[a]				
				Unabs.[b]	B. cell abs.[c]	GPK abs.[d]	B. cell abs.	GPK abs.			VCA[g]	EA[h]	IgM	NA	EBV Infection
Heterophil positive mononucleosis															
L. P.	19	6	MH+[i]	1792	112	1792	896	Pos.	7168	Pos.[j]	Pos.	320	40	80	<2	Recent inf.
A. G.	14	12	MH+	224	0	112	0	Pos.	56	Pos.	Pos.	160	80	80	20	Recent inf.
N. R.	2	6	MH+	28	0	14	0	Pos.	14	Neg.[k]	Pos.	10	<5	40	10	Recent inf.
Heterophil negative mononucleosis															
A. L. S.	2	2	MH-[l]	56	14	14	0	Pos.	224	Pos.	Pos.	10	<5	10	10	Recent inf.
		30		56	14	0	0	Pos.	56	Neg.	Pos.	20	<5	<10	20	
C. B.	5	20	MH-	28	7	0	0	Pos.	112	Pos.	Pos.	10	<5	80	2	Recent inf.
B. G.	31	25	MH-	56	14	56	0	Pos.	448	Pos.	Pos.	10	ND[m]	80	40	Recent inf.
Controls with recent EBV infection															
S. B.	6	No disease	C*[n]	28	7	0	28	Pos.	224	Neg.	Pos.	20	5	20	20	Recent inf.
M. M.	16	No disease	C*	14	0	0	0	Pos.	14	Neg.	Pos.	40	20	40	10	Recent inf.
Controls with past EBV infection															
D. M. P.	20	No disease	C*	28	7	14	0	Pos.	14	Neg.	Neg.	5	<5	<10	20	Past inf.
L. G.	23	No disease	C*	56	56	0	14	Pos.	28	Neg.	Neg.	20	<5	<10	40	Past inf.
Controls without EBV infection															
M. B. D.	11	No disease	C[o]	56	14	0	28	Neg.	28	Neg.	Neg.	<5			ND	None

[a]EBV, Epstein-Barr virus.
[b]Unabs., unabsorbed.
[c]B. cell abs., beef red cell absorbed.
[d]GPK abs., guinea pig kidney absorbed.
[e]MT, monotest (R).
[f]MS, monospot (R).
[g]VCA, viral capsid antigen.
[h]EA, early antigen.

[i]MH+, heterophil positive mononucleosis by sheep cells.
[j]Pos., positive test.
[k]Neg., negative test.
[l]MH-, heterophil negative mononucleosis by sheep cells.
[m]ND, not done; no serum left.
[n]C*, contact with a case of mononucleosis within 2 yr.
[o]C, control.

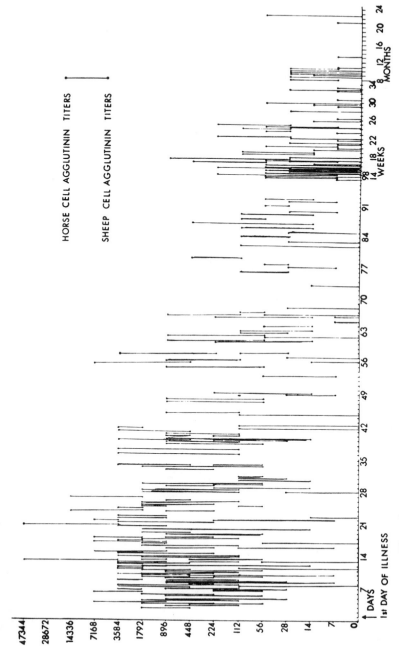

Figure 2. Horse cell and sheep cell agglutinin titers and lifespan in cases of infectious mononucleosis.

Table 4. Horse red blood cell agglutinins in slide tests in cases of infectious mononucleosis and in controls

Cases and sera	Horse cell agglutinins (slide test[a]) Monotest		
	Pos. sera	Neg. sera	Positive cases (%)
108 cases of mononucleosis with 244 sera	154 (83)[c]	12 (10)	89
93 cases with 169 het. pos.[b] sera	19 (18)	35 (25)	
with 56 het. neg. sera (in follow-up)			
15 cases with 19 het. neg. sera	11 (8)	6 (6)	75
280 controls with 304 sera (all het. neg.)	2 (2)	253 (238)	Less than 1

[a]A few tests could not be done because of insufficient amount of serum.
[b]Het. pos., heterophil positive; het. neg., heterophil negative. By Standard Paul Bunnell Davidsohn test with sheep cells.
[c]( ), no. of cases.

Table 5. Comparison of nonspecific heterophil agglutinins and specific EBV[a] antibodies in selected cases

Cases	Age (yr)	Days	Group	Sheep cell agglutinin titer			Horse cell agglutinin titer		MT[b]		MS[c]	EBV		
				Unabs.[d]	B. cell abs.[e]	GPK abs.[f]	B. cell abs.	GPK abs.	M[g]	m[h]		VCAA[i]	EA[j]	IgM
L.F.	14	84 days	MH+[k]	28	0	28	0	Pos. 56	−			40	20	
		128 days		28	0	7	7	Pos. 28				40	ND[l]	<5[m]
S.F.	11	61 days	MH+	28	0	28	7	Pos. 56	−	+	++	160	−	<5
G.H.	21	51 days	MH+	28	0	7	0	Pos. 28	−	+	+	20	−	<5
		71 days		28	0	7	0	Pos. 28	−	−	+	20	−	<5
P.L.	50	11 days	MH+	224	7	112	7	Pos. 448	−	+	++	40	5	5
H.L.	15	83 days	MH+	224	7	56	14	Pos. 224	−	+	+	320	−	5
M.P.	6	29 days	MH+	28	0	7	0	Pos. 56	−	+	++	320	−	<5
D.P.	21	57 days	MH+	56	0	14	ND		+	ND	ND	320		5
		71 days		0	0	0			−	−	−			
S.V.	8	No disease	C*[n]	14	0	0	7	Neg. 0	−	+	+	20	5	<5
C.S.	5	No disease	C*	ND	7	0	7	Neg. 0	−	−	−	40	5	<5
				ND			0	Neg. 0	−	−	−	40	<5	<5
C.T.	2½	No disease	C*	0	0	0	0	Neg. 0	−	−	−	40	<5	<5
				0	0		0	Neg. 0	−	−	−	40	<5	<5
C.B.	3	No disease	C*	14	7	0	0	Neg. 0	−	−	−	−	<5	<5
												−		<5

[a] EBV, Epstein-Barr virus.
[b] MT, monotest.
[c] MS, monospot (R).
[d] Unabs., unabsorbed.
[e] B. cell abs., beef red cell absorbed.
[f] GPK abs., guinea pig kidney absorbed.
[g] M, macroscopic agglutination.

[h] m, microscopic agglutination.
[i] VCA, viral capsid antigen.
[j] EA, early antigen.
[k] MH+, heterophil positive mononucleosis by sheep cells.
[l] ND, not done; no serum left.
[m] <5, negative at the stated dilution (light microscopic magnification 100×).
[n] C*, contact with a case of mononucleosis within 2 yr.

done; it was found to be positive, as for instance in case N. R. (Table 3), thereby confirming that the monotest was falsely negative in these cases.

In contrast (Table 6), the monospot test was positive in all cases of heterophil positive or heterophil negative mononucleosis. This slide test, however, gave a fine agglutination in almost half of the control cases and, since a negative control serum is not provided with the monospot test, it is difficult to determine when the test is to be considered negative. Again, the extremely long lifespan of the horse cell agglutinin may account for many of these apparently false positive monospot tests, probably many more than with the horse cell microtiter test since, on slide, the test is carried out on undiluted sera.

Specific EBV-VCA antibodies were found in virtually all cases of heterophil positive infectious mononucleosis and in 86% of heterophil negative cases (Table 7). These antibodies were found in only 67% of the controls, a prevalence which is in the range usually found in an unselected middle-age population.

The EBV-EA antibodies appeared in 43% of cases of heterophil positive mononucleosis and in 45% of heterophil negative cases (Table 8). In another published series (9), these antibodies could be demonstrated in up to 70% of cases. The diagnostic value of this test is further limited by the fact that detectable EA antibody titers have been found in up to 10% of control cases in our series. When a careful inquiry into the possibility of contact with a case resembling infectious mononucleosis was made, and when children were eliminated from the group, the prevalence of these antibodies in controls could be lowered to 5%, but this difference is not statistically significant. The lifespan of these antibodies, as a rule, was relatively short, but as shown in Figure 3, they have been found to last for over 12 months in many cases and for over 2 years in 7 cases.

The EBV-IgM antibodies have been measured in relatively few cases in our series to date. The relative prevalence of these antibodies in cases of heterophil positive mononucleosis, in heterophil negative cases, and in controls, is shown in Table 9. The appearance of these antibodies in controls in our series was associated with EBV seroconversion or with a significant rise in EBV antibodies. From our results to date, these antibodies appeared short-lived, lasting usually 2 months or less as shown in Table 10. In two cases (R. P. and J. B.) of mononucleosis thus far, however, the EBV-IgM antibodies reappeared approximately 1 year after the original disease, in association, at least in one of the two cases, with a mild mononucleosis-like syndrome. This observation is not too much of a surprise since definite IgM responses have been reported recently in the course of proved rubella (18, 19), herpes simplex reinfections (20), and also in herpes zoster (21).

In 4 of 11 cases of mononucleosis tested thus far, the EBNA antibodies appeared at least 1 month later than the EBV-VCA antibodies in the course of the disease (Tables 3 and 10). Henle et al. (15) reported similar results in a

Table 6. Horse red blood cell agglutinins in slide tests in cases of infectious mononucleosis and in controls

Cases and sera	Horse cell agglutinins (slide test[a]) monospot			
	Pos. sera	Doubtful sera (fine aggl.)	Neg. sera	Positive cases (%)
108 cases of mononucleosis with 244 sera				
93 cases with 169 het. pos.[b] sera	149 (76)[c]	20 (17)	0[d]	(100)
with 56 het. neg.[b] sera (in follow-up)	5 (5)	51 (51)	0	
15 cases with 19 het. neg. sera	8 (8)	10 (8)	–	(100)
280 controls with 304 sera (all het. neg.)	–[e]	174 (148)	122 (120)	(55)

[a] A few tests could not be done because of insufficient amount of serum.
[b] Het. pos., heterophil positive; het. neg., heterophil negative. By Standard Paul Bunnell Davidsohn test with sheep cells.
[c] ( ), no. of cases.
[d] 0, none found; all sera tested.
[e] –, none found among the available sera.

Table 7. EBV-VCA antibodies in cases of infectious mononucleosis and in controls

Cases and sera	Specific antibodies (indirect immunofluorescence) EBV-VCA[a] antibodies		
	Pos. sera	Neg. sera	Positive cases (%)
108 cases of mononucleosis with 244 sera			
93 cases with 169 het. pos.[b] sera	106 (90)[c]	3 (33)	(100)
with 56 het. neg. sera (in follow-up)	56 (43)	0[d]	
15 cases with 19 het. neg. sera	16 (12)	2 (2)	(86)
280 controls with 304 sera (all het. neg.)	146 (123)	155 (61)	(67)

[a]EBV-VCA, Epstein-Barr virus-viral capsid antigen.
[b]Het. pos., heterophil positive; het. neg., heterophil negative. By Standard Paul Bunnell Davidsohn test with sheep cells.
[c]( ), no. of cases.
[d]0, none found; all sera tested.

Table 8. Prevalence of EBV-EA[a] antibodies in heterophil positive and negative mononucleosis and in controls with and without contact with mononucleosis

	Cases No. positive/ total no. tested	%	Sera No. positive/ total no. tested
Het. pos. mono.[b]	45/85	53	98/198
Het. neg. mono.[c]	5/11	45	5/14
Controls			
Contacts of cases	8/73	10.9	9/95
No contact	3/58	5.2	3/152

[a]EBV-EA, Epstein-Barr virus-early antigen.
[b]Het. pos., heterophil positive mononucleosis by sheep cells.
[c]Het. neg., heterophil negative mononucleosis by sheep cells.

larger series of cases. The combination, therefore, of a positive EBV-VCA test and a negative EBNA test early in the course of infectious mononucleosis may be useful in the diagnosis of a certain number of cases of the disease. The EBV-IgM antibody test, however, will probably become the ideal diagnostic test, especially if combined with a negative EBNA test, since the possibility of EBV reactivation would thereby be eliminated.

CONCLUSION

The comparative analysis of specific and nonspecific test results in mononucleosis allows the following conclusions. Horse cell microtiter tests and the

Table 9. Prevalence of EBV[a]-IgM antibodies in heterophil positive and negative mononucleosis and in controls with and without contact with mononucleosis

	Cases No. positive/ total no. tested	%	Sera No. positive/ total no. tested
Het. pos. mono.[b]	14/14	100	22/39
Het. neg. mono.[c]	3/5	60	3/11
Controls			
Contact of cases	1/6	16	1/6
No contact	1/12	8	2/22

[a]EBV, Epstein-Barr virus.
[b]Het. pos., Heterophil positive mononucleosis by sheep cells.
[c]Het. neg., Heterophil negative mononucleosis by sheep cells.

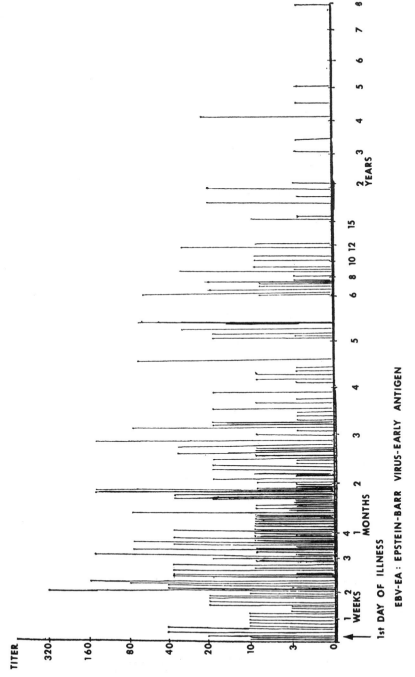

Figure 3. EBV-EA antibody titer and lifespan in cases of infectious mononucleosis.

Table 10. Time of appearance of EBNA antibodies compared to other antibodies in relation to onset of disease in selected cases of mononucleosis

Patient	Antibody	Time[a]							
		−2 mo	+2 wk	+1½ mo	3½ mo	5 mo	8 mo	18 mo	28 mo
S. O.	EBNA[b]	<2	<2	<2	20	20	40	20	40
	VCA[c]	<5	40	40	40	80	40	20	
	EA[d]	<5	<5	<5	<5	<5			
	HHA[e]		448	448	0	14		0	
	SHA[f]				0	14		0	
	MM[g]		++	++	++	-+	--	-+	--
	IgM	<5	80	80	<5	<5	<5	<5	<5

Patient	Antibody	Time[a]								
		−14 mo	−2 wk	+1 wk	1 mo	2 mo	3 mo	14 mo	23 mo	25 mo
R. P.	EBNA	<2	<2	40	80	80	80	80	80	80
	VCA	<5	<5	160	320	320	320	160	160	160
	EA	<5	<5	320	160	160	80	40	20	20
	HHA			7168	896		448	56	56	56
	SHA			7168	224	14	56	7	7	7
	MM	--	--	++	++	++	++	-+	-+	--
	IgM	<5	<5	80	40	5	<5	5	7	7

Continued.

Table 10. *Continued.*

Patient	Antibody	Time[a]				
		+1 wk	3 wk	1½ mo	2½ mo	23 mo
G. McS.	EBNA	<2	40	20	20	20
	VCA	<5	160	320	320	40
	EA		80	80	80	
	HHA		896	896		
	SHA		448	56	14	
	MM	--	++	++	++	--
	IgM	<5	40	40	<5	

Patient	Antibody	Time[a]								
		+1 wk	1 mo	2 mo	3 mo	6 mo	10 mo	10½ mo	23 mo	27 mo
J. B.	EBNA	40	2	2	10	20	20		20	10
	VCA	320	160	320	320	320	320		160	160
	EA	20	5	<5	<5	<5	<5		<5	
	HHA	3584	112	112	224	28	14			
	SHA	1792		112	7	14	14			
	MM	++	++	++	++	-+	-+		--	--
	IgM	10	40	<5	<5	<5	5	5	<5	<5

		+1 wk	1½ mo	3 mo	5 mo	7 mo	9 mo	21½ mo	34 mo	35 mo	50 mo
J. D.	EBNA		<2	2	20	10		40	40		20
	VCA	160	80	80	160	160	160	160	80		80
	EA	10	10	20	20	40		10	10	10	10
	HHA				448	14	28				
	SHA	1792	448	56	28	0	0				
	MM	++	++	+	++	++		-+	--	--	--

[a]Time, weeks or months preceding or following onset of disease.
[b]EBNA, Epstein-Barr nuclear antigen antibody titer.
[c]VCA, viral capsid antigen antibody titer.
[d]EA, early antigen antibody titer.
[e]HHA, horse red blood cell heterophil antibody titer (guinea pig kidney absorbed).
[f]SHA, sheep red blood cell heterophil antibody titer (guinea pig kidney absorbed).
[g]MM, monotest and monospot test.

124   Jean H. Joncas

monospot are more sensitive than sheep cell microtiter tests and the monotest. False negative results are occasionally seen with sheep cell microtiter
tests (cases A. L. S., C. B., and B. G., Table 3) and the monotest (case N. R.),
but not with the other two tests. More false positive results are probably seen
with the horse cell microtiter test and particularly with the monospot test,
although many presumably false positive tests undoubtedly result from the
persistence of agglutinins detectable by these sensitive tests following a
clinically apparent or inapparent mononucleosis months before. The test
may, nevertheless, be false in relation to the disease investigated at the time.
Finally, specific EBV-EA antibody tests, and particularly EBV-IgM antibody
tests, are useful in the diagnosis of selected borderline cases of mononucleosis
(cases N. R. and C. B., Table 3). The elimination of nonspecific fluorescence
by a simple absorption procedure carried out on the antihuman IgM reagent
will facilitate its use in the future. The combination of a positive EBV-IgM
antibody test with a negative EBNA test appears to be the most conclusive
diagnostic finding in a patient with this disease (case L. P., Table 3). In the
vast majority of cases of mononucleosis, however, the Paul Bunnell Davidsohn test, particularly if carried out with horse cells, remains the most reliable
and the most useful test in the diagnosis of infectious mononucleosis.

ACKNOWLEDGMENTS

This study was supported in part by a Federal Provincial Health Research
Grant no. 604-7-783, a Defense Research Board Grant no. 1880-08, and a
FCAC Grant from the Province of Quebec, Department of Education.

LITERATURE CITED

1. Davidsohn, I., and C. L. Lee. 1962. The laboratory in the diagnosis of
infectious mononucleosis. Med. Clin. N. A. 46:225–244.
2. Joncas, J. 1972. The clinical significance of the EBV infection in man.
Progr. Med. Virol. 14:200–240.
3. Hoff, G., and S. Bauer. 1965. A new rapid slide test for infectious
mononucleosis. J. A. M. A. 194:351–353.
4. Lee, C. L., F. Zandrew, and I. Davisohn. 1968. Horse agglutinins in
infectious mononucleosis. Am. J. Clin. Path. 49(1):3–11.
5. Evans, A. S., J. C. Niederman, and R. W. McCollum. 1968. Seroepidemi-
ology studies of infectious mononucleosis with EB virus. New England J.
Med. 279:1121–1127.
6. Niederman, J. C., R. W. McCollum, and G. Henle. 1968. Infectious
mononucleosis. Clinical manifestations in relation to EB virus antibodies. J.
A. M. A. 203:205.
7. Joncas, J., and C. Mitnyan. 1970. Serological response of the EBV
antibodies in pediatric cases of infectious mononucleosis and in their
contacts. Canad. M. A. J. 102:1260–1263.

8. Joncas, J., J. C. Gilker, and A. Chagnon. 1974. Limitations of immuno-fluorescence tests in the diagnosis of infectious mononucleosis. Canad. M. A. J. 110:793–802.

9. Henle, G., W. Henle, and G. Klein. 1971. Demonstration of two distinct components in the early antigen complex of EBV infected cells. Internat. J. Cancer 8:272–282.

10. Henle, W., G. Henle, and J. C. Niederman. 1971. Antibodies to early antigens induced by Epstein-Barr virus in infectious mononucleosis. J. Infect. Dis. 124:58–67.

11. Banatvala, J. E., J. M. Best, and D. K. Waller. 1972. Epstein-Barr virus specific IgM in infectious mononucleosis, Burkitt lymphoma and naso-pharyngeal carcinoma. Lancet I (7762):1205–1208.

12. Schmitz, H., and M. Scherer. 1972. IgM antibodies to Epstein-Barr virus in infectious mononucleosis. Arch. ges. Virusforsch. 37:332–339.

13. Schmitz, H., D. Uslz, and C. Krainick-Reichert. 1972. Acute Epstein-Barr virus infections in children. Med. Microbiol. Immunol. 158:58–63.

14. Joncas, J., L. Chicoine, R. Thivierge, and M. Bertrand. 1974. EBV antibodies in the CSF of a case of infectious mononucleosis with encepha-litis. Am. J. Dis. Child. 127:282–285.

15. Henle, G., W. Henle, and C. A. Horwitz. 1974. Antibodies to Epstein-Barr virus-associated nuclear antigen in infectious mononucleosis. J. Infect. Dis. 130:231–239.

16. Reedman, M., and G. Klein. 1973. Cellular localization of an Epstein-Barr virus (EBV)-associated complement-fixing antigen in producer and non-producer lymphoblastoid cell lines. Internat. J. Cancer 11:499–520.

17. Ankerts, J., P. Christensen, L. Kjellen, and G. Kronvall. 1974. A routine diagnostic test for IgA and IgM antibodies to rubella virus: absorption of IgG with staphylococcus aureus. J. Infect. Dis. 130:268–273.

18. Ogra, P. L., D. Kerr-Grant, and G. Umana. 1971. Antibody response in serum and nasopharynx after naturally acquired and vaccine-induced infec-tion with rubella virus. New England J. Med. 285:1333–1338.

19. Strannegard, O., S. E. Holm, and S. Hermodsson. 1970. A case of apparent reinfection with rubella. Lancet I:240–241.

20. Nahmias, A., S. L. Shore, and I. Delbuono. 1974. Diagnosis by immuno-fluorescence of human viral infections with emphasis on herpes simplex infections. Comparative Immunodiagnosis of Viral Infections. Academic Press, New York.

21. Ross, C. A. C., and R. McDaid. 1972. Specific IgM antibody in serum of patients with herpes zoster infections. Brit. M. J. IV:522–523.

CHAPTER 11

Laboratory Diagnosis of the Autoimmune Diseases

Noel R. Rose

The body is endowed with astute and proficient mechanisms for distinguishing "self" from "nonself." The modern practice of blood transfusion depends upon the certainty that an individual with group A antigen on his tissue and blood cells will not form anti-A, even though he would produce anti-B if properly stimulated. Similarly, transplantation of solid organs, such as kidneys, has been made feasible by the recognition of surface alloantigens, the HL-A series, which distinguish human beings. Recipients given kidneys closely similar or identical in their HL-A antigens show better acceptance than those given poorly matched organs. These widely used procedures of blood transfusion and organ transplantation bear witness to the general validity of the rule of immunological self-recognition.

There is always a chance of breakdown of the controls underlying self-recognition, resulting in the appearance of autoimmune disease. Autoantibodies, or factors with antibody-like properties reacting with antigens of the individual himself, provide the key to the study of the autoimmune diseases, even though the antibodies may not produce the disease. The term "autoimmune disease" is generally reserved for those maladies in which immunological processes contribute significantly to the pathogenesis of the

The preparation of this chapter was aided by Public Health Service research grants CA 02357 and CA 16426 from the National Cancer Institute.

disease. But there are many other diseases in which the immunological response is secondary to the initial tissue injury. Autoantibodies may be of equal value in the diagnosis of these diseases.

The selection of a method for demonstrating autoantibodies is determined by the position and properties of the antigen and by the level of sensitivity desired. A few kinds of cells, especially erythrocytes, can be obtained in stable suspensions and lend themselves to agglutination tests. Soluble serum proteins can be used in precipitation or latex fixation tests. The most widely applicable method for studying antibodies to tissue antigens is indirect immunofluorescence, a procedure by which a patient's serum is applied to a frozen section of human or animal tissue containing the appropriate antigen. Fluorescein-labeled antiglobulin, or an antiserum specific for an individual immunoglobulin class, is then added to the washed tissue section to reveal specific localization of the patient's antibody. Autoantibodies to antigens of the blood or to the basement membranes of kidney, lung, or skin may localize in vivo, and their presence can be signaled by direct reaction with fluorescein-labeled antiglobulin in the case of tissue antigen, or agglutination by antiglobulin sera in the case of erythrocytes. Sometimes demonstration of localized complement is useful as an indicator of antigen-antibody reactions, as is a decrease in levels of circulating complement components.

Autoantibodies, as well as most autoimmune diseases, are more frequent in older ages. Some investigators have suggested that they represent a response to degraded or effete tissue components liberated during normal wear and tear. Others propose that an accumulation of somatic mutations in the immunological apparatus account for the rise in autoimmune reactions during aging. To the laboratory worker, this frequency of autoantibodies in the aging population is a warning that the demonstration of autoantibody by itself is not synonomous with the diagnosis of autoimmune disease.

Immunologists and clinicians differ in their requirements for accepting a human disease as autoimmune in origin. Clinically, a disease of unknown etiology with evidence of autoantibody formation is sometimes termed "autoimmune." Since patients may respond to immunosuppressive therapy, this definition has a pragmatic basis. A stricter set of criteria was proposed by us several years ago as a guide for current and future research (1). They include demonstration of antibodies or cell-mediated immunity operative under conditions of the body. The responsible antigen should be defined and isolated and used to engender an immunological response in experimental animals. Finally, pathological changes should appear in the corresponding tissue of the immunized that are similar to those seen in the human disease.

The essential feature of these criteria is the simulation of human disease by experimental immunization. This goal has been accomplished with certain diseases associated with organ-specific antigens. These diseases are characterized by chronic inflammation of a single organ corresponding to the responsible antigen. Other diseases seem to involve several organ systems and different antigens. In these cases, certain genetically determined disorders provide useful experimental models. Viral infection is related to the pathogenesis of some of these diseases. Information derived from the study of experimentally induced and genetically determined autoimmune diseases have proved to be of great value in understanding human autoimmune diseases.

AUTOANTIBODIES IN HUMAN DISEASE

In Table 1 are given some of the most prominent human diseases associated with autoantibody production. They are arranged as a spectrum from the strictly organ specific autoimmune diseases to more generalized disorders. There is a tendency for more than one autoimmune disease to occur in the same individual. The overlap is usually within the same region of the spectrum. The patient may have more than one autoimmune disease of the endocrines, such as thyroiditis and adrenalitis, or more than one connective tissue disease, such as Sjogren's syndrome (keratoconjunctivitis sicca) and lupus. In addition, there is a significantly higher incidence of autoantibodies to other organ-specific antigens in patients with one autoimmune disease. For example, 25% of thyroiditis patients have antibody to gastric parietal cells, while 45% of patients with pernicious anemia have antibody to one of the antigens of thyroid (2, 3). Twenty-five percent of patients with Addison's disease have antibody to thyroid (3) as do 20% of patients of diabetes mellitus (4), suggesting that in these endocrine diseases, also, there may be some autoimmune factor. The aggregation of autoimmune responses to immunologically distinct organ-specific antigens is best explained as a genetic idiosyncracy comparable to atopy in the immediate hypersensitivity reactions.

Autoantibodies are often present in the sera of normal individuals, as described previously. The incidence is closely related to age and sex. For example, the incidence of autoantibodies to thyroglobulin is about 3% in males and 15% in females less than 30, while in 50- to 70-year-old subjects, it amounts to 15% in men and 35% of women (5). The incidence of antinuclear antibodies is biased in a similar manner, so that over 20% of women aged 60 or more are positive (6, 7). These observations suggest a role of sex hormones, together with an accumulation of genetic errors in production of the autoimmune response.

ENDOCRINE DISEASES

Autoantibodies to thyroglobulin are most easily demonstrated by means of the tanned cell hemagglutination test (8). Indirect immunofluorescence is also applicable provided the human or monkey thyroid tissue used as substrate has

Table 1. Principal autoimmune diseases

Disease	Antigen	Detection of autoantibody
Chronic thyroiditis (Hashimoto's disease and primary myxedema)	Thyroglobulin	Precipitation
		Hemagglutination
		Latex fixation
		Immunofluorescence
	Microsome	Complement fixation
		Immunofluorescence
	CA$_2$	Immunofluorescence
	Surface membrane	Cytotoxicity
		Mixed agglutination
Hyperthyroidism	Surface membrane	Bioassay (LATS)
Adrenal insufficiency (Addison's disease)	Microsome of the adrenal cortex	Immunofluorescence
		Hemagglutination
Primary hypoparathyroidism	Oxyphilic cells	Immunofluorescence
	Principal cells	Immunofluorescence
Pernicious anemia and atrophic gastritis	Microsomes of parietal cells	Immunofluorescence
		Complement fixation
	Intrinsic factor	Radioimmunoassay

Orchitis and masculine infertility	Spermatozoa	Agglutination Cytotoxicity Immunofluorescence
Lens-induced uveitis	Crystallin	Precipitation Delayed hypersensitivity
Sympathetic ophthalmia	Uveal pigment	Hemagglutination Immunofluorescence
Pemphigus vulgaris	Intracellular substance of stratified squamos epithelium	Immunofluorescence
Bullous pemphigoid	Basement membrane of stratified squamous and columnar epithelium	Immunofluorescence
Myasthenia gravis	Striations of skeletal and heart muscle	
Autoimmune glomerulorephritis (Goodpasture's syndrome)	Glomerular basement membrane of kidney and lung	Immunofluorescence (linear pattern)
Immune complex glomerulonephritis	Tubular epithelium and brush border Nuclear components	Immunofluorescence (granular pattern)

Continued.

Table 1. *Continued.*

Disease	Antigen	Detection of autoantibody
Primary biliary cirrhosis	Mitochondria (distal tubular cells of kidney)	Immunofluorescence Complement fixation
Chronic active hepatitis	Smooth muscle (gastric mucosa) Nuclei	Immunofluorescence Immunofluorescence
Idiopathic thrombocytopenic purpora	Platelets	Platelet survival Antiglobulin consumption Mixed agglutination Lysis Complement fixation
Acquired hemolytic anemia	Erythrocytes	Antiglobulin Anticomplement
Ulcerative colitis	Colonic cells Colonic lipopoly-saccharide	Cytotoxicity Hemagglutination
Keratoconjunctivitis sicca (Sjogoen's disease)	Salivary ducts	Immunofluorescence
	Thyroglobulin Nuclei	(See chronic thyroiditis) (See systemic lupus)
Scleroderma	Nucleoli	Immunofluorescence

Disease	Component	Method
Dermatomyositis	Nuclear components	Immunofluorescence
Systemic lupus erythematosus (LE)	Whole nuclei	LE test
	Single stranded DNA	Immunofluorescence
	Native DNA	Precipitation
	Extractable nuclear antigen (ENA)	Complement fixation
	Acidic nuclear protein (Sm)	Hemagglutination
	Nucleoprotein	Radioimmunoassay
	RNA nucleotides	
	Mitochondria	Complement fixation
	Microsomes	Complement fixation
Rheumatoid arthritis	Immunoglobulin	Latex fixation
		Sensitized sheep cell agglutination
		Rh agglutination
		Precipitation
		Hemagglutination
	Collagen	Anti-globulin consumption

been fixed with methanol to prevent the thyroglobulin from leaking out during washing (9). In our experience, 65% of patients with nonspecific chronic thyroiditis have significant titers (> 10) of antibody, and regularly titers of > 1000. Patients with most other forms of thyroiditis have lower percentages and low titers (10). However, patients with primary, spontaneous myxedema also have the same high incidence and high titers of autoantibodies to thyroglobulin as thyroiditis patients (10, 11).

Thyroglobulin autoantibodies can be measured by other commonly used serological techniques, such as precipitation or latex fixation (12, 13). They fail, however, to give positive complement-fixation reactions. There is a second, unrelated antigen of thyroid extracts responsible for complement-fixation by 70% thyroiditis sera (14). It is associated with the microsomal fraction of epithelial cells, especially those from stimulated or hyperplastic thyroids. The fluorescent antibody test is also useful for measuring antibody to thyroid microsomes, employing unfixed sections of human or monkey tissue as substrate.

While most patients with thyroiditis have both thyroglobulin and microsomal autoantibodies, some have one and not the other. Putting together all thyroiditis patients with one or both autoantibodies, one finds 90% to 99% positive, so that negative serological tests virtually exclude thyroiditis. On the other hand, about 20% of patients with adenocarcinoma of the thyroid have antibodies to thyroid antigens, so that a positive test does not rule out thyroid cancer (9).

In the presence of complement, the sera of many thyroiditis patients prevent suspensions of primate thyroid cells from attaching to the walls of a culture vessel (15). These so-called cytotoxic antibodies are directed to a component of the thyroid surface membrane as shown by the mixed agglutination reaction. The antibodies are frequent in both chronic thyroiditis and myxedema, and seem to be especially prevalent in juvenile goiter (9).

Some antibodies to the thyroid surface may stimulate, rather than damage, the cells. Long-acting thyroid stimulators (LATS), which are found in many cases of thyroid hyperplasia or thyrotoxicosis (Graves' disease), cause prolonged (24-hr) hyperactivity of the mouse thyroid, contrasting with the short-term (2-hr) stimulation produced by thyroid-stimulating hormone (16, 17). It is believed that LATS is responsible for the transient hyperthyroidism sometimes seen in the newborn infant of a thyrotoxic mother. The activity can be absorbed by human thyroid microsomes (18). Some hyperthyroid sera that do not have LATS activity in the mouse bioassay block the ability of human thyroid microsomes to absorb LATS, an activity called "LATS protector."

Autoantibodies to cortical cells are encountered in about one-half of the cases of idiopathic adrenal insufficiency (Addison's disease) (19, 20) and in a very much smaller proportion of patients with tuberculous Addision's disease

(20). Antibodies to cells with steroid-synthesizing granules seem to occur in some cases of premature menopause (21). When present, antibodies to the steroid-secreting cells cross-react with the analogous cells in ovary, testes, and placenta (22). Primary hypoparathyroidism is found in 20% of adrenalitis patients, along with the appropriate autoantibodies. Rather common in children is the co-existence of candidiasis with hypoparathyroidism, Addison's disease, and, less often, thyroid disease or pernicious anemia (23).

There is a striking parallel between the immunological findings in pernicious anemia and chronic thyroiditis. Antibodies to the gastric parietal cells, like those to the thyroid epithelial cells, are demonstrable by complement-fixation and indirect immunofluorescence, and react with microsomes (24). Equivalent to the autoantibodies to thyroglobulin are circulating or secretory agents that combine with intrinsic factor (25). Some antibodies block the combination of cobalamine (B-12) with intrinsic factor while others co-precipitate with the B-12-intrinsic factor complex. If radioactive B-12 is used, binding antibody can be precipitated with the complex by half-saturated ammonium sulfate and the radioactivity in the precipitate counted. Blocking activity, on the other hand, can be assayed by determining the amount of uncombined B-12 absorbed by activated charcoal.

SPERM

Antibodies to spermatozoa can be tested by agglutination in a dilute gelatin medium, and by immobilization or cytotoxicity in the presence of complement. Fresh sperm suspensions must be used for these procedures. Immunofluorescence tests using methanol-fixed sperm have also been described (26). The antibodies are found in about 10% of men with unexplained infertility as well as in about half of men with accidental or deliberate interruption of the spermatic ducts (e.g., vasectomy) (27). The antibodies seem to impede the movement of sperm through cervical mucus. Women may also have antibodies to sperm, but their significance is not understood at this time.

RENAL DISEASES

Experimentally, it is possible to induce antibodies to the glomerular basement membrane which produce typical signs of glomerulonephritis (28–31). The antibodies attach to the basement membranes of kidney and, sometimes, lung in vivo, as demonstrated by linear staining with the appropriate fluorescent antiglobulin reagent. In a small percentage of human cases of glomerulonephritis (Goodpasture's syndrome), a similar pattern of labeled antiglobulin localization is found in kidney biopsies (32). In addition to immunoglobulins, the third component of complement (C3) is deposited in a linear pattern (32). It is likely that these antibodies actually localize in kidney (and perhaps lung) of the patient and produce tissue damage by activating complement.

In most kidney biopsies obtained from human cases of glomerulo-nephritis, immunoglobulins and C3 are found as irregular deposits along the epithelial side of the glomerular basement membrane (33). This granular pattern of localization is characteristic of experimental or clinical serum sickness attributable to formation of antigen-antibody complexes in slight antigen excess (34). Sometimes it is possible to elute the immunoglobulin from nephritis kidneys and show that they are antibodies to nucleotides (as in lupus nephritis), the renal tubular epithelium, or the renal brush border (35, 36). Often no particular antigen can be implicated, although circumstantial evidence suggests that antigens of microorganisms, such as β-hemolytic strep-tococci, are responsible.

A common feature of both forms of immunological glomerulonephritis is a lowered level of circulating complement (37, 38). Measurement of total complement or of some individual components may have prognostic value.

BLOOD DISEASES

On a clinical basis, the extrinsic hemolytic anemias can be divided into those associated with warm antibodies, active at body temperature, and cold antibodies, which combine with erythrocytes only at lowered temperatures (39). An antiglobulin (Coombs) reagent can be used to demonstrate that erythrocytes are coated with IgG in most cases of warm antibody hemolytic anemia (40). Sometimes antibody to C3 will also react (40). Warm antibody hemolytic anemia may be primary (idiopathic) or secondary to underlying malignant or autoimmune disease. On occasion, the IgG, eluted from the patient's erythrocytes by gently heating, has detectable antibody activity against one of the antigens of the Rh system, such as "e" (41, 42). Cold antibodies of hemolytic anemia are generally IgM, but anti-C3 serves as an effective antiglobulin reagent (43–45). The eluted antibody often has speci-ficity for blood group antigens I or i (46). This form is commonly associated with *Mycoplasma* pneumonia, infectious mononucleosis, or lympho-proliferative disease (43, 47). The biphasic hemolysin of Donath and Land-steiner (48) is found after viral or syphilitic infection, and gives erythrocyte eluates with anti-P or -p activity (49).

In many cases of idiopathic thrombocytopenic purpura, antibody to the platelets are probably involved. The peculiar surface properties of platelets make the antibodies difficult to demonstrate reliability with the usual sero-logical tests, and in vivo survival is often resorted to. Sometimes the antibody is directed to a drug rather than the platelet itself, so that serum of the patient will lyse the platelet only in the presence of drugs. The reaction requires complement.

CONNECTIVE TISSUE DISEASE

About 75% of patients with rheumatoid arthritis have demonstrable rheumatoid factors (50). In addition, a third of patients with lupus, Sjogren's syndrome, and chronic active hepatitis, as well as a few individuals with chronic infections, have these factors (50). The major characteristic of the rheumatoid factors is their ability to react with the Fc portion of aggregated IgG. The antigen is usually fixed to latex particles in the form of purified human gamma globulin (F II) or to sheep erythrocytes as a subagglutinating dose of rabbit antibody. Rh positive cells coated with human anti-D may also be employed. Most of the rheumatoid factors are in the IgM class, but IgG rheumatoid factors are not infrequent. Occasionally they may complex in vivo. Aggregates can be found in the synovial fluids by precipitation in the cold or with Clq. Immunoglobulin complexes with complement are taken up by phagocytic macrophages in the synovial membranes (51). They probably lead to release of lysosomal enzymes which contribute to the arthritis. Low levels of complement in the joint fluid, therefore, are indicative of active disease (52, 53). Antibodies to degraded collagen are also present in rheumatoid sera, but their pathogenetic significance is unknown.

In systemic lupus erythematosus (LE), one sees an astonishing array of auto-antibodies to nuclear components, cytoplasmic constituents, erythrocytes, platelets, clotting factors, and aggregated IgG (54–56). In addition, many patients have positive serological tests for syphilis. Of special diagnostic value is the presence of LE cells in peripheral blood or marrow of about 70% of cases (57). The cells represent the phagocytosis by polymorphonuclear neutrophils of cellular nuclei opsonized by antinuclear antibody and complement. The antigen is probably found on the nuclear membrane, but can be absorbed by native DNA protein (57). There are many other antinuclear factors even more frequent than the LE factor itself. The usual test for antinuclear antibodies (ANA) is carried out by indirect immunofluorescence using young rat or mouse liver sections as substrate, but imprints of spleen or even films of peripheral leukocytes have been used in some laboratories. Virtually all lupus patients (98 to 100%) are positive, as are some patients with rheumatoid arthritis, scleroderma, and dermatomyositis (58). Some definition of the nuclear antigen involved can be obtained from the pattern of localization. For instance, the nucleolar and speckled patterns are distinctive and often associated with diffuse scleroderma (59). Other separate antinuclear factors can be extracted and tested by standard immunological procedures such as radioimmunoassay, hemagglutination, or complement-fixation. The most prevalent antibodies in lupus sera are directed to single-stranded DNA (87%), then to native DNA (60%), while fewer sera react with synthetic polynucleotides (60). Nuclear antigens extractable in neutral or in acid buffers (Sm and ENA) are also being used and have a certain prognostic value (61, 62).

SUMMARY

The demonstration of autoantibodies is important in many diseases of unknown etiology. The appropriate immunological procedure depends upon the position and location of the antigen. Antibodies to cell surface antigens of blood cells or spermatozoa can be detected by agglutination, cytotoxicity, immobilization, or lysis. Antiglobulin procedures are often useful for demonstrating nonagglutinating antibodies. Soluble serum proteins or tissue extracts lend themselves to precipitation, passive agglutination, or complement-fixation. The most widely applicable method for studying antibodies to tissue antigens, without having to extract them, is indirect immunofluorescence. The pattern of localization often presents information about the nature of the antigen. Be they primary or secondary, pathogenic or harmless, autoantibodies provide valuable diagnostic clues in many human diseases.

LITERATURE CITED

1. Witebsky, E., N. R. Rose, K. Terplan, J. R. Paine, and R. W. Egan. 1957. Chronic thyroiditis and autoimmunization. J. A. M. A. 164:1439.
2. Doniach, D., I. M. Roitt, and K. B. Taylor. 1963. Autoimmune phenomena in pernicious anemia: Serological overlap with thyroiditis, thyrotoxicosis and systemic lupus erythematosus. Brit. M. J. 1:1374.
3. Irvine, W. J., S. H. Davies, S. Teitelbaum, I. W. Delamore, and A. W. Williams. 1965. The clinical and pathologic significance of gastric parietal cell antibody. Ann. New York Acad. Sci. 124:657.
4. Whittingham, S., J. D. Mathews, I. R. Mackay, A. E. Stocks, B. Ungar, and F. I. R. Martin. 1971. Diabetes mellitus, autoimmunity, and aging. Lancet 1:763.
5. Doniach, D., and I. M. Riott. 1969. Autoimmune thyroid disease. In P. A. Miescher and H. J. Muller-Eberhard (eds.), Textbook on Immunopathology, Vol. II, pp. 516–533. Grune & Stratton, Inc., New York.
6. Seligmann, M., A. Cannat, and M. Hamard. 1965. Studies on antinuclear antibodies. Ann. New York Acad. Sci. 124:816.
7. Svec, K. H., and B. C. Veit. 1967. Age-related antinuclear factors: Immunologic characteristics and associated clinical aspects. Arthritis Rheum. 10:509.
8. Fulthorpe, A. J., I. M. Roitt, D. Doniach, and K. G. Couchman. 1961. A stable sheep cell preparation for detecting thyroglobulin autoantibodies and its clinical applications. J. Clin. Path. 14:654.

9. Rose, N. R., and E. Witebsky. 1968. Thyroid autoantibodies in thyroid disease. *In* R. Levine and R. Luft (eds.), Advances in Metabolic Disorders, Vol. 3, pp. 231–277. Academic Press, Inc., New York.

10. Witebsky, E., and N. R. Rose. 1963. Autoimmunity and its relationship to thyroid disease. N. Y. State J. Med. 63:56.

11. Anderson, J. W., W. M. McConahey, D. Alarcon-Segovia, R. F. Emslander, and K. G. Wakim. 1967. Diagnostic value of thyroid antibodies. J. Clin. Endoc. 27:937.

12. Roitt, I. M., D. Doniach, P. N. Campbell, and R. V. Hudson. 1956. Autoantibodies in Hashimoto's disease (lymphadenoid goiter). Lancet 2:820.

13. Doniach, D. Thyroid autoimmune disease. 1967. J. Clin. Path. 20: (Suppl.) 385.

14. Belyavin, G., and W. R. Trotter. 1959. Investigations of thyroid antigens reacting with Hashimoto sera: Evidence for an antigen other than thyroglobulin. Lancet 1:648.

15. Pulvertaft, R. J. V., D. Doniach, and I. M. Roitt. 1961. The cytotoxic factor in Hashimoto's disease and its incidence in other thyroid disease. Brit. J. Exper. Path. 42:496.

16. Adams, D. D., and H. D. Purves. 1956. Abnormal responses in the assay of thyrotoxin. Proc. Univ. Otaga Med. School 34:11.

17. McKenzie, J. M. 1968. Humoral factors in the pathogenesis of Graves' disease. Physiol. Rev. 48:252.

18. Beall, G. N., and D. H. Solomon. 1966. Inhibition of long acting thyroid stimulator by thyroid particulate fractions. J. Clin. Invest. 45:552.

19. Blizzard, R. M., R. W. Chandler, M. Kyle, and W. Hung. 1962. Adrenal antibodies in Addison's disease. Lancet 2:901.

20. Goudie, R. B., J. R. Anderson, K. K. Gray, and W. G. Whyte. 1966. Autoantibodies in Addison's disease. Lancet 1:1173.

21. Irvine, W. J., M. M. W. Chan, L. Scarth, F. O. Kolb, M. Hartog, R. I. S. Baylis, and M. I. Drury. 1968. Immunological aspects of premature ovarian failure associated with idiopathic Addison's disease. Lancet 2:883.

22. Irvine, W. J. 1971. Adrenalitis, hypoparathyroidism, and associated diseases. *In* M. Samter (ed.), Immunological Diseases, Vol. II, p. 1218. Little, Brown & Company, Boston.

23. Blizzard, R. M. 1969. Idiopathic hypoparathyroidism: A probable autoimmune disease. *In* P. A. Meischer (ed.), Textbook of Immunopathology, Vol. II, p. 548. Grune & Stratton, Inc., New York.

24. Chanarin, I. 1968. The stomach in allergic diseases. *In* P. G. H. Gell and R. R. A. Coombs (eds.), Clinical Aspects of Immunology, p. 1024. F. A. Davis Company, Philadelphia.

25. Jeffries, G. H., D. W. Hoskins, and M. H. Sleisenger. 1962. Antibody to intrinsic factor in serum from patients with pernicious anemia. J. Clin. Invest. 41:1106.

26. Hjort, T., and K. B. Hansen. 1971. Immunofluorescent studies on human spermatozoa. I. The detection of different spermatoxoae antibodies and their occurrence in normal and infertile women. Clin. Exper. Immunol. 8:9.

27. Rumke, P. The spermatozoa and testes in allergic disease. 1969. *In* P. G. H. Gell and R. A. Coombs (eds.), Clinical Aspects of Immunology, p. 1152. F. A. Davis Company, Philadelphia.

28. Cavelti, P. A., and E. S. Cavelti. 1945. Studies on the pathogenesis of glomerulonephritis. III. Clinical and pathologic aspects of the experimental

glomerulonephritis produced in rats by means of autoantibodies to kidney. Arch. Path. 40:163.

29. Hunter, J. L. P., D. B. Hackel, and W. Heymann. 1960. Nephrotic syndrome in rats produced by sensitization to rat kidney proteins: Immunologic studies. J. Immunol. 85:319.

30. Steblay, R. W. 1962. Glomerulonephritis induced in sheep by injections of heterologous glomerular basement membrane and Freund's complete adjuvant. J. Exper. Med. 116:253.

31. Steblay, R. W. 1963. Glomerulonephritis induced in monkeys by injections of heterologous glomerular basement membrane and Freund's adjuvant. Nature, London 197:1173.

32. Duncan, D. A., K. N. Drummond, A. F. Michael, Jr., and R. L. Vernier. 1965. Pulmonary hemorrhage and glomerulonephritis: Report of six cases and study of the renal lesion by fluorescent antibody technique and electron microscopy. Ann. Int. Med. 62:920.

33. Feldman, J. D., M. R. Mardiney, and S. E. Shuler. 1966. Immunology and morphology of acute post-streptococcal glomerulonephritis. Lab. Invest. 15:283.

34. Dixon, F. J. 1962–1963. The role of antigen-antibody complexes in disease. Harvey Lect. 58:21.

35. Edington, T. S., R. J. Glassock, and F. J. Dixon. 1968. Autologous immune complex nephritis induced with renal tubular antigen. I. Identification and isolation of the pathogenetic antigen. J. Exper. Med. 127:555.

36. Andres, G. A., L. Accinni, S. M. Beiser, C. L. Christian, G. A. Cinotti, B. F. Erlanger, K. C. Hsu, and B. C. Seegal. 1970. Localization of fluorescein-labeled antinucleoside antibodies in glomeruli of patients with active systemic lupus erythematosus nephritis. J. Clin. Invest. 49:2106.

37. Lange, K., and L. B. Slobody. 1960. Significance of serum complement levels for diagnosis and prognosis of acute and sub-acute glomerulonephritis and lupus erythemotosus disseminatus. Ann Int. Med. 53:636.

38. West, C. D., A. J. McAdams, J. M. McConville, N. C. Davis, and N. C. Holland. 1965. Hyposcomplementemic and normocomplementemic persistent (chronic) glomerulonephritis: Clinical and pathological characteristics. J. Pediat. 67:1089.

39. Leddy, J. P., and S. N. Swisher. 1971. Acquired immune hemolytic disorders. In M. Samter (ed.), Immunological Disease, Vol. II., p. 1097. Little, Brown & Company, Boston.

40. Leddy, J. P. 1966. Immunological aspects of red cell injury in man. Seminars Hemat. 3:48.

41. Leddy, J. P., P. Peterson, M. A. Yeaw, and R. F. Bakemeier. 1970. Patterns of serologic specificity of human γG erythrocyte autoantibodies. J. Immunol. 105:677.

42. Dacie, J. V. 1962. The haemolytic anaemias, congenital and acquired: Part III. The autoimmune Haemolytic Anaemias. 2nd Ed. Grune & Stratton, Inc., New York.

43. Capra, J. D., P. Dowling, S. Cook, and H. G. Kunkel. 1968. Cold reactive antibodies in infectious mononucleosis: Delineation of an incomplete γG antibody with I specificity. Clin. Res. 16:300.

44. Goldberg, L. S., and E. V. Barnett. 1967. Mixed γG-γM cold agglutination. J. Immunol. 99:803.

45. Harboe, M., H. J. Müller-Eberhard, H. Fudenberg, M. J. Polley, and P. L. Mollison. 1963. Identification of the components of complement participating in the antiglobulin reaction. Immunology 6:412.

46. Marsh, W. L. 1961. Anti-i: A cold antibody defining the Ii relationship in human red cells. Brit. J. Haemat. 7:300.

47. Liu, C., M. D. Eaton, and J. T. Heyl. 1959. Studies on primary atypical pneumonia: II. Observations concerning the development and immunological characteristics of antibody in patients. J. Exper. Med. 109:545.

48. Donath, J., and K. Landsteiner. 1904. Ueber paroxysmale Hamoglobinurie. München med. W-chn-schr. 51:1590.

49. Worlledge, S. M., and C. Rousso. 1965. Studies of the serology of paroxysmal cold haemoglobinuria (P.C.H.) with special reference to its relationship with P blood group system. Vox Sang. 10:293.

50. Mackay, I. R., and F. M. Burnet. 1963. Autoimmune Diseases. Charles C Thomas, Publisher, Springfield, Ill., p. 141.

51. Rawson, A. J., N. M. Abelson, and J. L. Hollander. 1965. Studies on the pathogenesis of rheumatoid joint inflammation. II. Intracytoplasmic particulate complexes in rheumatoid synovial fluids. Ann. Int. Med. 62:281.

52. Winchester, R. J., V. Agnello, and H. G. Kunkel. 1969. The joint-fluid γG-globulin complexes and their relationship to intra-articular complement diminution. Ann. New York Acad. Sci. 168:195.

53. Ruddy, S., and K. F. Austen. 1970. The complement system in rheumatoid synovitis. I. An analysis of complement component activities in rheumatoid synovial fluids. Arthritis Rheum. 13:713.

54. Holman, H. R. 1960. The LE cell phenomenon. Ann. Rev. Med. 11:321.

55. Kunkel, H. G., and E. Tan. 1965. Autoantibodies and disease. Advances Immunol. 4:351.

56. Symposium on immunologic aspects of rheumatoid arthritis and systemic lupus erythematosus. 1963. Arthritis Rheum. 6:402.

57. Holman, H. R., and H. R. Deicher. 1959. The reaction of the lupus erythmatosus (L. E.) cell factor with deoxyribonucleoprotein of the cell nucleus. J. Clin. Invest. 38:2059.

58. Friou, G. J. 1958. Clinical application of a test for lupus globulin-nucleohistone interaction using fluorescent antibody. Yale J. Biol. & Med. 31:40.

59. Burnham, T. K., and P. W. Bank. 1974. Antinuclear antibodies. I. Patterns of nuclear immunofluorescence. J. Invest. Dermat. 62:526.

60. Koffler, D., R. Carr, V. Agnello, R. Thoburn, and H. G. Kunkel. 1971. Antibodies to polynucleotides in human sera. Antigenicity specificity and relation to disease. J. Exper. Med. 134:294.

61. Sharp, G. C., W. S. Irvin, R. L. LaRoque, C. Velez, V. Daly, A. D. Kaiser, and H. R. Holman. 1971. Association of autoantibodies to different nuclear antigens with clinical patterns of rheumatic disease and responsiveness to therapy. J. Clin. Invest. 50:350.

62. Reichlin, M., and M. Mattioli. 1972. Correlation of a precipitin reaction to an RNA protein antigen and a low provalence of nephritis in patients with systemic lupus erythematosus. New England J. Med. 286:908.

SECTION IV

New Trends in Methodology in Laboratory Microbiology

Introduction

Kenneth R. Cundy

As this symposium has progressed, it has become obvious that many new and refined procedures are becoming available for the microbiologist-scientist to choose as valuable aids for rapid and specific laboratory diagnosis. Application of some time-honored, as well as newly developed techniques, for the detection and identification of microbial antigens and/or their products of metabolism has made this goal reasonably attainable. As more and more laboratories begin to incorporate these newer methods into their routine battery of microbiological and immunological tests, it has become even more obvious that the accumulation of additional data at a more rapid rate demands, in many instances, a sophisticated delivery and storage system for results. This, in turn, has generated much interest in computerization. Whereas our colleagues in clinical chemistry laboratories have applied computerization for many years, it is only in the past 5 years that progress has been made by the microbiology laboratory.

The detection of hepatitis B antigen (HB_sAg) in serum by the use of solid-phase radioimmunoassay has become familiar to most laboratories as a sensitive and convenient technique. There are many other acceptable applications of this technique in microbiology and other laboratories involved in performing diagnostic tests for the presence of microbial and other compounds. As an example, one of the newest and most interesting applications of radioimmunoassay is that for identification of *Herpesvirus hominis* in tissue cultures infected with clinical materials. It is to this subject of radio-immunoassay and its myriad applications in the field of competetive protein binding that Dr. Fleisher will address himself.

A more rapid detection of microbial growth from clinical specimens became technically feasible with the application of radiometric techniques to a blood culture system. This system has been widely tested and extensively discussed during the past 5 years and the application of it to quality control for microbial contamination and other tests involving detection and/or inhibition of metabolism has become of paramount interest to many microbiologists. Dr. Randall will comment on the level of accuracy and proficiency which this sytem has attained in her experience. Her comments should further stimulate the intense interest in this area.

Similarly in the same time period, a little over 5 years ago, Dr. Cherry, together with Dr. C. Wayne Moss, provided us with prophetic food for thought in their editorial which appeared in the *Journal of Infectious Diseases* on the role of gas chromatography in the clinical microbiology laboratory. I quote their concluding sentence, "Gas chromatography is a powerful and versatile analytical tool capable of producing such large amounts of significant data that its invasion of the clinical microbiology laboratory is inevitable." At that time, publication experience in microbiological fields only extended back about 6 years. In the ensuing 5 years, much has been accomplished in this exciting field, whether it be the application of gas-liquid chromatography to the analysis and detection of bacterial products or metabolites or to the analysis of their cellular chemical composition. Even more exciting is the prospect of analyzing body fluids for such compounds, thus bypassing or at least augmenting the culture system. Dr. Mandle will further define this subject, drawing upon his work together with that of Dr. Thomas Wade.

Dr. Kunz will draw upon his extensive experience with computerization in the microbiological context. In his laboratory, man and machine are attempting to augment and integrate the information provided by rapid and precise laboratory methods. Dr. Kunz's application of automation and computerization to the determination and delivery of antimicrobial susceptibility tests results is well known and should provide us with a valuable insight into the state of the art.

CHAPTER 12

Radioimmunoassay as Applied to Microbiology

Martin Fleisher

Our interest in the specific area of radioimmunoassay procedures applicable to microorganism analysis was initiated by an evaluation of the diagnostic efficacy of urinary carcinoembryonic antigen (CEA) (1). The possible spurious elevation in CEA concentration, due to urinary tract infection in patients with bladder and prostatic carcinoma required investigation and clarification. Kass (2) first defined bacteriuria as being associated with a colony count of more than 100,000 bacteria/ml. Others have indicated that quantitative cultures are the best laboratory procedure for documenting the presence of urinary tract infection (3, 4). Since many patients with neoplastic disease of the bladder are subject to bladder infection, the problem of nonspecific interference in the clinical evaluation of CEA was studied. Ten different strains of three groups of Gram negative microorganisms usually found in high count were tested for CEA assay interference. These were *Escherichia coli, Klebsiella pneumoniae,* and *Proteus mirabilis.* Table 1 summarizes the results of this investigation. Fortunately, our concern was proved unwarranted. However, it was this investigation which initiated our interest in immunological testing for microbiological organisms. Our belief then and now is that the immunological approach to microbiological analysis is the real future for this discipline.

Fundamentally, the specifications for immunomicrobiological analysis should include the following: (a) provide a rapid and specific diagnosis; (b) yield reliable results; and (c) provide for ease of quantitation.

Table 1. Results of simulated urinary tract infection with three commonly encountered species of Gram negative rods

Organism	Number of strains $(10^5$ organisms/ml)	Effect on CEA assay
Escherichia coli	10	Undetectable
Klebsiella pneumoniae	10	Undetectable
Proteus mirabilis	10	Undetectable

What is described above, in simple terms, are the requirements for acceptable radioimmunoassay procedures for measurement of *any* compound. An excellent review of RIA principles and methods has been published (5).

Under appropriate conditions, and if care is taken to obtain a pure antigen preparation and subsequently a specific antibody, the technique of RIA offers the following keystones for a good clinical diagnostic tool: specificity, accuracy, and precision. It appears, however, that there are two main drawbacks or obstacles to the development of RIA and competitive protein binding (CPB) as applied to microbiology. The first is a lack of antigenic specificity for specific organisms. This of course obviates the specifications of *specificity* and *accuracy*. The second obstacle has been the frequency with which more than one specific organism is involved in the causative role of a disease. The latter counteracts the precision and efficiency of the assay procedure for diagnostic purposes.

Notwithstanding these obstacles, the progress of RIA technology in microbiology has been recognized for its vast potential. Significant inroads have been made into the development of this field. A brief review of the state of immunoassay procedures for microorganism analysis will substantiate this point.

The developmental interests have been approached from two points of view. One deals with the microorganisms for which immunological techniques involve the antigenicity of the polysaccharide and lipoprotein components of bacterial cell walls or antigens attached to bacterial cell walls. The second approach deals with specific antigens elaborated by the microorganisms. For example, the antigenic polysaccharide chain, of the 08 antigen of *E. coli,* has been elucidated (6). The polysaccharide moiety of the lipopolysaccharide from *E. coli* F492 (08: K27−: H−) and the polysaccharide from the rfa mutant F612 (derived from F492) were isolated by extraction with 45% aqueous phenol at 65°. The results of this analysis are shown in Table 2. Based on these analyses, it seems probable that the polysaccharide sequence contains approximately 20 repeating units of α-mannosyl-1, 2-α-mannosyl-1, 2-α-mannose which are joined by α-1, 3-linkages.

These data represent more information than we presently have for many of the antigens being measured and associated with different disease states. A

Table 2. 08 antigen of *E. coli* (polysaccharide analysis) (6)

Constituents	% (Based on dry bacteria)	
	E. coli F492	*E. coli* F612
Mannose	83.5	99.2
Glucose	5.7	—
Galactose	3.4	—
Heptose	4.6	—
2-keto-3-deoxy-mannosulonic acid	0.8	—
Molecular weight	12,400	10,400

variety of organisms have been successfully measured with the use of two basic techniques: RIA and radioimmunological assay.

Table 3 summarizes a few recent and important contributions of RIA application to microorganism analysis which includes assays for viral antigens, antiviral antibodies, plant viruses, as well as various bacterial organisms.

Hutchinson and Ziegler (8) developed a simplified, indirect radioimmunoassay for *E. coli,* vaccinia virus, and herpesvirus. The antigens of these microorganisms were affixed to glass cover slips. The antigen-antibody reaction takes place directly on the cover slip and the unbound antiserum is easily separated from the bound antiserum by rinsing the cover slip with water. Rabbit or human immune serum were reacted with the antigens and the primary immune complex were quantitated by a secondary reaction with ^{125}I-labeled globulin (antirabbit or antihuman). A direct relationship between the antiserum concentration and the ^{125}I absorption was estab-

Table 3. Immunoassay techniques for microorganisms

Organism	Assay procedure	Investigators (reference no.)
Plant viruses *E. coli*	Solid phase RIA	Ball (7)
Vaccinia Virus Herpes Virus	RIA	Hutchinson and Ziegler (8)
E. coli	Radioimmunological assay	Brown and Lee (9)
Staphylococcal enterotoxins A and B	Solid phase RIA	Johnson, Bukovic, and Kauffman (10)
Type A toxin of *Clostridium botulinum*	RIA	Boroff and Su-Chen (11)
Pneumococcal polysaccharide	RIA	Kenny et al. (12)
Viral antigens and antiviral antibody	Solid phase micro RIA	Rosenthal, Hayashi, and Notkins (13)

lished. This affords an objective, quantitative evaluation of antibody and the results were reported to be reproducible.

Boroff and Shu-Chen (11) have applied RIA techniques for the measurement of type A toxin of *Clostridium botulinum*. A preparation of pure type A toxin of botulinum was labeled with ^{131}I. The radioactive toxin was used in a radioimmunoassay according to the procedure of Berson and Yalow (14). Dilutions of antibody relative to the toxin, capable of binding 50% of the added ^{131}I toxin, were mixed with a sample of labeled toxin and various concentrations of unlabeled toxin. A standard curve was established that could be used to determine the concentration of cold toxin in a test mixture. This assay was sensitive to 100 mouse minimum lethal dose and was highly specific for the serological type of the toxin used. Kenny et al. (12) were able to detect type-specific pneumococcal polysaccharide (types 1, 2, 3, 4, 5, 8, 12, and 18) in serum from bacteremic patients using the technique of immunoelectroosmophoresis with rabbit anticapsular antibody. The assay was sensitive to 0.2 ng/ml of polysaccharide type, a factor of 10 times more sensitive than immunodiffusion. In a correlation study of 46 patients, 12 out of 20 bacteremic patients with pneumonia showed antigenemia. No circulating antigen was detected in 26 patients negative for bacteremia. Although this procedure is far from ideal, in terms of its concordance with bacterial culture, it does offer the advantage of rapid diagnosis and type-specific diagnosis within approximately 1 hour. It is interesting to note that Bukantz, deGara, and Bullawa (15) reported a higher proportion of deaths in patients with antigenemia (60%) than in bacteremia without antigenemia (14%).

Brown and Lee (9) reported the use of a radioimmunological method for the quantitative measurement of naturally occurring human serum antibodies reactive with *E. coli*. The method was shown to be sensitive to 5 ng of antibody nitrogen, specific, and quantitative. This procedure is based on the primary binding of IgG, IgA, and IgM to a nonenteropathogenic strain of *E. coli* and secondary reaction with radiolabeled rabbit antihuman immunoglobulins. Anti-*E. coli* antibodies were measured in sera of 11 healthy subjects and 72 patients with immunological or gastrointestinal disorders.

The technique of counterimmunoelectrophoresis (CIE) was used by Fossieck, Graig, and Paterson (16) for the rapid diagnosis of meningitis due to *Diplococcus pneumonia*. Serum, urine, and cerebrial spinal fluid were assayed for antigens of *Diplococcus pneumonia* and correlated well with Gram stain examination (Table 4). Pneumococcal antigen was present in the body fluids from five of the six patients. Sequential analyses of specimens from individual patients revealed striking variations in persistance of antigen in CSF and in serum and urine as well. The capacity of CIE to yield a definitive diagnosis of pneumococcal infection has obvious diagnostic advantage. This technique is sensitive to nanogram concentrations of antigen and a definitive diagnosis can be obtained within 1 hr. In dealing with suspected bacterial meningitis, speed of diagnosis is essential for the initiation of rational treatment and management of the patient.

Table 4. Detection of antigen from *Diplococcus pneumoniae* (16)

Patient	Antigen detected by CIE				
	CSF	Serum	Urine	Serotype	CSF Gram stain
A	+	+	+	8	+
B	+	+	+	8	+
C	+	+	+	17	+
D	+	NT^a	NT	3	0
E	+	NT	NT	23	0
F	0	0	NT	–	+

^{a}NT denotes not tested.

Current emphasis on guidelines for microbiology centers around such problems as productivity in the microbiological laboratory, microbiological utilization in the small hospital, test cost factors, specimen quality control, proficiency testing, and whether or not speciation is as essential as heretofore believed. Many of these problems are not unique to microbiologists. The clinical chemist is also concerned with test volume and costs, as well as quality control and proficiency testing. However, the common denominator for all clinical laboratory disciplines is test efficiency and accuracy. The clinical chemist has begun to close the gap on these problems and I suspect the microbiologist is experiencing the same progress. Perhaps the approach to microbiological analysis discussed above will help to achieve these goals. Radioimmunoassay applied to microbiology will eliminate costly unnecessary work as well as provide information of greater clinical relevance.

LITERATURE CITED

1. Fleisher, M., H. Grabstald, F. Mamaril, H. Oettgen, C. Pinsky, W. F. Whitmore, and M. K. Schwartz. 1974. Urinary carcinoembryonic antigen levels in patients with cancer. Clin. Chem. 20:864.
2. Kass, E. H. 1956. Asymptomatic infection of the urinary tract. Tr. A. Am. Physicians 69:56–64.
3. Kaitz, A. L., and E. J. Williams. 1960. Bacteriuria and urinary tract infection in hospitalized patients. New England J. Med. 262:425–430.
4. Kunin, C. M., E. Zacha, and A. J. Paquin, Jr. 1962. Urinary tract infection in school children. I. Prevalence of bacteriuria and associated urologic findings. New England J. Med. 266:1287–1296.
5. Skelly, D. S., L. P. Brown, and P. K. Besch. 1974. Radioimmunoassay. Clin. Chem. 19:146–186.
6. Reske, K., and K. Jann. 1972. The 08 antigen of *Escherichia Coli*. Structure of the polysaccharide chain. European J. Biochem. 31:320–328.
7. Ball, E. M. 1973. Solid phase radioimmunoassay for plant viruses. Virology. 55:516–520.

8. Hutchinson, H. D., and D. W. Ziegler. 1972. Simplified radioimmuno-assay for diagnostic serology. Appl. Microbiol. 24:742−749.

9. Brown, W. R., and E. M. Lee. 1973. Radioimmunologic measurements of naturally occurring bacterial antibodies. 1. Human serum antibodies reactive with *Escherichia Coli* in gastrointestinal and immunologic disorders. J. Lab. Clin. Med. 82:125−136.

10. Johnson, H. M., J. A. Bukovic, and P. E. Kauffman. 1973. Staphylococcal enterotoxins A and B: Solid-phase radioimmunoassay in food. Applied Microbiol. 26:309−313.

11. Boroff, P. A., and G. Shu-Chen. 1973. Radioimmunoassay for type A toxin of *clostridium botulinum*. Appl. Microbiol. 25:545−549.

12. Kenny, G. E., B. B. Wentworth, R. P. Beasley, and H. M. Foy. 1972. Correlation of circulating capsular polysaccharide with bacteremia in pneumococcal pneumonia. Infect. Immunity 6:431−437.

13. Rosenthal, J. D., K. Hayaski, and A. L. Notkins. 1973. Comparison of direct and indirect solid-phase microradioimmunoassays for the detection of viral antigens and antiviral antibody. Applied Microbiol. 25:567−573.

14. Berson, S. A., and R. S. Yalow. 1957. Kinetics of reaction between insulin and insulin-binding antibody. J. Clin. Invest. 36:873−881.

15. Bukantz, S. C., P. F. deGara, and J. G. M. Bullawa. 1942. Capsular polysaccharide in the blood of patients with pneumococcic pneumonia. Arch. Int. Med. 69:191−212.

16. Fossieck, B., Jr., R. Graig, and P. Y. Paterson. 1973. Counter immunoelectrophoresis for rapid diagnosis of meningitis due to diplococcus pneumonia. J. Infect. Dis. 127:106−109.

CHAPTER 13

Radiometric Techniques in Microbiology

Eileen L. Randall

Radiometric methodology has been utilized in a variety of microbiological techniques. These include detection of bacteremia, determination of microbial susceptibility, detection of bacteria in food, bacterial identification and differentiation, detection of white cell metabolism, and sterility testing.

BACTEREMIA

DeLand and Wagner (1) first reported the use of a medium containing ^{14}C-glucose to detect early bacterial growth in blood. More than 100 organisms of 15 species were studied and all produced detectable quantities of $^{14}CO_2$. Little release of $^{14}CO_2$ was noted during the first 4 to 6 hr of incubation, but, after this time, it was released in large quantities. The release of $^{14}CO_2$ was related to the pH of the medium and agitation of the culture medium resulted in earlier release.

An automated radiometric method for detection of bacteremia capable of handling 10 cultures simultaneously was described by DeLand and Wagner (2). One hundred forty simulated and 500 actual blood cultures were examined by this method. No microorganisms were encountered that did not produce CO_2 from the metabolism of glucose. The average time to detect the presence of bacteria in the simulated cultures was less than 4 hr and the maximum time was 6 hr. Thirty positive and no false negative or false positive cultures were obtained in the 500 blood cultures from patients. In four cases, organisms were detected by the radiometric method that were not found by routine bacteriological procedures.

DeBlanc, DeLand, and Wagner (3) compared the automated radiometric instrument, BACTEC, which handles 25 samples simultaneously, with conventional methods in the detection of bacteremia. A total of 2,967 cultures from 1,280 patients were studied. Of 57 patients positive by one or both methods, conventional techniques detected bacteria in 87% and the radiometric method detected bacteria in 85%. Seventy percent of the cultures were detected first by the radiometric method, 65% of these on the day of innoculation. In 8 cultures where radiometric detection was negative but subcultures were positive, a microaerophilic streptococcus was isolated. Failure of the organism to metabolize glucose was probably related to the aerobic conditions used in the study. Washington and Uy (4), however, concluded that the radiometric method lacked the sensitivity required for a suitable alternative to conventional techniques. They investigated 59 simulated blood cultures and 65 blood cultures from patients with suspected bacteremia. In their simulated blood cultures containing between 4 and 4,250 organisms/ml, they were unable to detect bacterial growth within 6 hr, but in their next testing interval, 12 hr later, growth was detected in all of 13 cultures containing *Staphylococcus aureus,* all of 14 cultures containing *Escherichia coli,* 13 of 17 cultures containing *Pseudomonas aeruginosa,* and 10 of 15 cultures containing group D streptococci. They reported negative results in some patients with bacteremia due to *P. aeruginosa,* group D streptococci, and *Bacteroides fragilis.* Only aerobic conditions were utilized which would explain the inability to detect *B. fragilis.*

Renner, Gatheridge, and Washington (5) compared the detection of bacteremia utilizing the automated BACTEC system with a conventional two-bottle system. Of 1,445 blood cultures, 106 were positive by both methods. The conventional system yielded 85 and the BACTEC yielded 84 positive cultures. The radiometric system failed to detect 22 cultures which were positive by the conventional method and the conventional method failed to detect 21 cultures positive by the BACTEC system. The BACTEC system had a slight advantage over the conventional system in the time interval required for detection. However, the recovery rates and detection times of anaerobes were less efficient by the BACTEC than by the conventional system.

A comparison of the BACTEC radiometric method with a routine method utilizing Columbia broth in detecting bacteremia due to aerobic organisms showed that of 1,261 blood cultures examined, 311 had significant results (6). This high rate of positivity (25%) was probably due to the fact that 42% of the patients with positive blood cultures were in the hospital burn unit where blood was drawn daily. BACTEC detected 91% of positive cultures as compared with 88% detected by the conventional method. Fifty-nine percent were detected by BACTEC, 11% were detected first by the conventional method, and 30% required the same time for detection by both methods.

In comparing the automated BACTEC system with the B-D vacutainer culture tube method, Smith and Little (7) found the radiometric method much more efficient. Of 105 positive cultures from 1,194 blood specimens, 92% were detected radiometrically, while 55% were detected by the conventional method. Forty-five percent were detected by BACTEC only, 48% were detected by both methods, and 8% were detected by the conventional method only.

Caslow, Ellner, and Kiehn (8) compared the BACTEC system with blind subculture for detection of bacteremia. Aerobic, anaerobic, and hypertonic vials containing an experimental Columbia broth rather than the standard tryptic soy broth were used in the study. Aerobic vials were read at 3-hr intervals up to 24 hr. Anaerobic and hypertonic vials were read at 16 to 24 hr and all vials were reread at 48 hr and at 7 days. Subcultures of aerobic and hypertonic bottles were made at 24 hr and 7 days. Subcultures of anaerobic bottles were made at 48 hr and 7 days. In 1,000 blood cultures, 104 isolates were recovered from 97 patients. All organisms recovered on subcultures were eventually detected by BACTEC. Seventy-eight percent of the aerobic positives and 81% of the hypertonic positives were detected by 24 hr. Three of the aerobic positive bottles which were not radiometrically detected at 24 hr had companion bottles which did detect at 24 hr. One hundred percent of the aerobic vials and 99% (all but 1 isolate) of the hypertonic vials gave positive growth indices at 48 hr.

The automated BACTEC was compared to a conventional system utilizing BD blood culture bottles containing trypticase soy and thioglycollate broths (9). Of 2,622 blood cultures examined, 226 (105 patients) were positive by one or more methods. The conventional system detected 4% more positive cultures than did BACTEC, but the mean detection time of BACTEC was calculated to be 1.48 days as compared with 2.18 days for the conventional system. The radiometric system required 50% less technician's time than the conventional system.

In a study on the radiometric detection of bacteremia in neonates, the predicted prevalence of false positive blood cultures due to hyperactive neonatal blood cells was confirmed (10). The suppression of this blood background radioactivity was achieved by using the hypertonic medium containing 10% sucrose. The aerobic 6A and high sucrose 4A bottles were utilized in the BACTEC system. These bottles were tested when they arrived in the laboratory, at 10 hr when possible, and daily for 7 days. The radiometric system produced accurate results as fast as the conventional method (brain heart infusion broth), saved labor, and minimized the recovery of extraneous contaminants.

The BACTEC system for detection of bacteremia has been used by Randall (11, 12) since December 1972 in two separate institutions, one a large 670-bed university teaching institution, the other a 500-bed community hospital. At the first institution, in comparing the automated BACTEC system with the conventional system consisting of a BD trypticase soy broth and Difco thiol broth, the BACTEC system detected 84% and the conventional system 75% of 144 significant isolates from 1,530 blood cultures. The two systems were comparable in detecting Enterobacteriaceae and nonfermenting gram-negative rods. However, the BACTEC system was more efficient in detecting staphylococci, yeast, and anaerobes, while the conventional system detected more streptococci. The BACTEC system detected bacteremia much more rapidly than did the conventional system. In the conventional system, an automatic 24-hr subculture system was utilized. Approximately 50% of Enterobacteriaceae, 24% of nonfermenting Gram negative rods, 24% of streptococci, 32% of staphylococci, and 6% of miscellaneous organisms were detected by BACTEC in 12 hr or less. Fifty-one percent of all aerobic organisms were detected by 24 hr. The conventional system usually required 48 hr for significant information to be obtained.

The BACTEC system detects bacteremia most rapidly when caused by members of the Enterobacteriaceae, pseudomonads, and staphylococci, the organisms which comprise up to 60 to 70% of the positive cultures in most hospitals. Median detection times of 13 to 16 hr for 133 isolates of Enterobacteriaceae and 53 isolates of *S. aureus* and 17 to 20 hr for 67 isolates of pseudomonads were obtained.

In the second institution, where the BACTEC system has been in use since June 1974, a modification has been made which results in even more rapid detection of positive specimens. All blood cultures from the previous day, including those logged in up to 7 a.m. of the present day, are rechecked at 2 p.m. Many positives are picked up at this time which come from blood cultures incubating at times less than 24 hr. Another innovation is the use of a shaking incubator which shakes all cultures even after they have been removed from BACTEC.

False positive results were a problem in the early use of the radiometric system, but, subsequently, have been of little concern. False negatives have occurred most commonly when streptococci are involved, but the author feels that no cases of infection have been missed when due to streptococci, as at least one bottle from a series of cultures has detected the organism.

The effect of osmotic stabilizers on $^{14}CO_2$ production by bacteria and blood was reported by Zwarun (13). A control medium was the aerobic 6A BACTEC culture vial containing 30 ml of tryptic soy broth plus ^{14}C substrate. Hypertonic media consisted of control medium with 1 and 3% NaCl, 10% sucrose, and 5, 10, and 15% dextran. Evolution of $^{14}CO_2$ by whole blood as well as by pneumococci, *Haemophilus* species, *Pseudomonas* species, and *Streptococcus pyogenes* was examined using the BACTEC system. Three percent NaCl was most deleterious to bacterial growth. It appeared from the studies that 10% sucrose was the most useful osmotic agent for the radiometric technique. Even though $^{14}CO_2$ production was lowered with this agent, blood $^{14}CO_2$ also was lowered.

An evaluaton of the efficacy of a ^{14}C-labeled osmotically stabilized (OS) blood culture medium in an automated BACTEC blood culture system has been done (14). The OS medium was compared to a similar tryptic soy broth that lacked 10% sucrose and was used with an anaerobic culture bottle. Of 78 aerobic or facultative organisms isolated, 67 were isolated from the OS medium, 61 in the aerobic medium, and 62 in the anaerobic medium. The OS medium failed to detect 7 pneumococci and 3 *Klebsiella,* while the aerobic medium did not detect 5 *E. coli,* 6 *Klebsiella,* 1 pneumococcus, 2 *H. influenzae,* and 1 *S. pyogenes.* The BACTEC OS medium appears to be slightly superior to the standard aerobic culture medium when used in conjunction with the anaerobic medium, since most pneumococci are readily isolated in the anaerobic medium. Inability to recover the pneumococci from the OS medium may be due in part to the high acidity produced by pneumococci in media which is stabilized with sucrose.

A comparison of macroscopic, microscopic, and radiometric examinations of clinical blood cultures in hypertonic media was reported by Rosner (15). Three bottles of BACTEC 8A medium containing tryptic soy broth with 10% sucrose were inoculated. One was examined only visually, one only microscopically, and one by BACTEC. All bottles were examined 4, 8, 16, 24, 36, and 48 hr after collection of the specimen and subcultured after incubation for 48 hr. Of 360 blood cultures found to contain organisms by subculture, 334 were first detected by BACTEC, 98 by macroscopic examination, and 68 by microscopic examination. By the end of 24 hr of incubation, BACTEC had detected 313 (93%) of those cultures eventually found to be positive. The author explained the low rate of positive findings of the macroscopic and microscopic methods on the basis of the cloudiness in the hypertonic medium which develops within 12 to 24 hr. BACTEC gave 11 false positive, the macroscopic, 75, and the microscopic, 35. BACTEC failed to detect 3 *Candida* species, 2 *Bacteroides,* 6 *Enterococcus,* 1 *Haemophilus,* and 1 *Neisseria* during the 48-hr incubation period.

SUSCEPTIBILITY TESTING

Metabolic inhibition as an index of bacterial susceptibility to drugs was reported by DeLand (16). The inhibition of glucose metabolism by antibiotics was evaluated based on radiometric methodology utilizing BACTEC. The susceptibility to drugs was determined within several hours after inoculation of the cultures. There is a consistent relationship between dose-response curves determined by the inhibition of glucose metabolism and minimal inhibitory concentrations (MIC) determined by a serial broth dilution technique.

Other investigators reported similar results on the automatic radiometric measurement of antibiotic effect on bacterial growth utilizing BACTEC (17). The antibiotic effect on bacterial growth was standardized by measuring the evolution of $^{14}CO_2$ 3 hr after inoculation. In 50 of 179 experiments (28%), each testing one organism against serial concentrations of an antibiotic, the concentration of antibiotic producing a 50% reduction of $^{14}CO_2$ within 3 hr after inoculation in comparison with a control culture was the same as the MIC determined by the broth dilution technique. In 129 experiments (72%), the antibiotic concentrations inhibiting $^{14}CO_2$ release to 50% of the control level were less than the MIC values. In testing strains of penicillinase producing S. aureus against penicillin, early suppression of $^{14}CO_2$ released cannot be used as evidence of sufficient antibiotic effect for clinical purposes.

BACTERIA IN FOOD

The radiometric technique has been used for detection of food-borne bacteria (18). *Salmonella typhimurium* and *S. aureus* detection times ranged from 10 to 3 hours for inocula of 10^0 to 10^4 cells/ml of broth when inoculated into tryptic soy broth containing 0.0139 μCi of ^{14}C-glucose/ml of medium. Heat-shocked spores of *Clostridium sporogenes* and *C. botulinum* require 3 to 4 hr longer for detection than comparable numbers of aerobic vegetable cells. Organisms were also inoculated into beef loaf and detection times were 2 hr for 5×10^4 salmonellae inoculated/ml of tryptic soy broth supplemented, 4 hours for 3×10^4 staphylococci, 5 hr for 4×10^5 *C. sporogenes* spores, and 5 to 6 hr for 10^6 *C. botulinum* spores. Thus, rapid detection by the radiometric method of organisms commonly associated with food contamination or spoilage was shown to be possible.

Later, Previte, Wells, and Rowley (19) reported on further modifications of the same medium to permit detection of nonfermentors of glucose using pseudomonads and *Alcaligenes faecalis*. Substrates screened for $^{14}CO_2$ production included uniformly labeled ^{14}C-glucose and pyruvate, 5-^{14}C and 1-^{14}C glutamate, 1-^{14}C lactate, and ^{14}C formate. Of the pseudomonads, *P. diminuta* was most difficult to detect rapidly.

BACTERIAL IDENTIFICATION

Camargo et al. (20) reported on the development of a radiometric technique based on the use of an ionization chamber to measure the $^{14}CO_2$ produced by bacterial metabolism of ^{14}C-substrates by mycobacterial strains. Utilizing 5 ml of liquid Middlebrook 7H9 (ADC additive) containing 2 μCi of ^{14}C-acetate or ^{14}C-glycerol, detection of significant bacterial metabolism of *Mycobacterium tuberculosis* within 18 hr (10^6 organisms inoculum) was possible. *Mycobacterium lepraemurium* produced readily detectable $^{14}CO_2$ when inoculated into 10 ml of a simple buffer medium (K-36) or a complex nutrient medium (NC-5). Although *M. lepraemurium* did not divide in the media, they have shown that it was metabolically active. Both organisms metabolized ^{14}C-acetate to $^{14}CO_2$ more rapidly than ^{14}C-glucose. They stated that the radiometric technique shows promise as a rapid and efficient system for detecting and determining drug susceptibilities of *M. tuberculosis* and *M. lepraemurium.*

Larson et al. (21) utilized BACTEC to detect the inhibition of carbohydrate metabolism of groups A, B, C, and D streptococci and group C *Salmonella* by streptococcal and *Salmonella* antisera. The inhibition is type-specific for *Salmonella,* as group E *Samonella* are inhibited only by *Salmonella* E antiserum and not by A or C_1 *Salmonella* antisera. Major cross-reactivity for streptococci occurs. At high concentrations, the antisera are bactericidal, but at more dilute concentrations, carbohydrate metabolism is suppressed. The radiometric technique is more sensitive than the capillary flocculation or visual detection of bacterial growth for detecting the inhibition of streptococci and salmonellae by specific antibodies. Specific antisera for bacterial species identification may be used in an automated system for detection of bacterial growth.

WHITE CELL METABOLISM

A radiometric screening test has been used for chronic granulomatous disease (22). Flasks containing 1-^{14}C-glucose and latex particles or Hank's balanced salt solution are inoculated with heparinized whole blood. After 1-hr incubation with shaking at 37°C, $^{14}CO_2$ production was measured on BACTEC. Little $^{14}CO_2$ production was detected in the resting samples without latex, irrespective of the number of phagocytic cells present. In the samples containing latex, readings were higher and dependent on the number of cells added. When 10^6 phagocytes were present, BACTEC readings were all above 30. Three known male children with chronic granulomatous disease were assayed by the method. Results of the radiometric (BACTEC) assay compared favorably with the liquid scintillation assay of hexose monophosphate shunt activity and effectively discriminated these subjects from normal samples. In addition, these authors demonstrated the effect of polyanethol sulfonate, a polyanionic anticoagulant, on leukocyte hexose monophosphate shunt activity. There was a dose-related effect with obliteration of the phagocytic hexose monophosphate shunt stimulation at high concentrations of polyanethol sulfonate. With the level of polyanethol sulfonate in blood culture bottles at 0.05%, white cell activity was significantly impaired.

A radiometric screening test of cell-mediated immunity based on phytohemagglutinin (PHA)-induced changes in lymphocyte carbohydrate metabolism was reported by Larson, Merz, and Wagner (23). They developed a rapid radiometric technique based on measurement of $^{14}CO_2$ produced by metabolism of ^{14}C-glucose using an ionization chamber to quantitate the radioactivity. PHA induced a marked change in lymphocyte carbohydrate metabolism within 1 hr after addition to the test system and peak stimulation occurred within 2 hr. The authors felt the radiometric technique held promise as an important improvement in the assessment of the response of the lymphocyte to PHA, as most other tests useful in assessing immune competence currently in use take from 3 to 7 days.

MISCELLANEOUS TECHNIQUES

Other applications of the radiometric BACTEC system reported by Waters and Zwarun (24) include testing the sterility of radiopharmaceuticals, frozen blood and blood components, and process water for a brewery.

Future developments in the use of the radiometric method include *Neisseria* differentiation, gentamicin serum assay, and urine screening. The use of radioactive glucose, maltose, and fructose to differentiate *N. gonorrhaeae* and *N. meningitidis* from other *Neisseria* species is being investigated (J. R. Waters, personal communication). Lactose is not used since it gives false positives and is volatile. Ortho-nitrophenyl-beta-galactopyranoside (ONPG) can be utilized for a rapid test for lactose fermentation. A heavy inoculum is used, incubated for 3 hr and read radiometrically. A negative test gives a less than 10 growth index on BACTEC, while a positive gives greater than 50. More than 100 species have been tested with 100% correlation. Also under development is a 2-hr serum assay for gentamicin, utilizing a radiometric technique. When utilizing the radiometric system for bacteriuria, various problems have been encountered. Significant bacteriuria due to members of the Enterobacteriaceae and enterococci can be determined within several hours, but cannot be determined when caused by pseudomonads. For this reason, the radiometric detection of significant numbers of organisms in urines in hospital laboratories is probably not practical, but may be applicable to screening urines in outpatient clinics, such as maternity clinics where *Pseudomonas* is not a problem.

LITERATURE CITED

1. DeLand, F. H., and H. N. Wagner, Jr. 1969. Early detection of bacterial growth with carbon-14-labeled glucose. Radiology 92:154–155.
2. DeLand, F. H., and H. N. Wagner, Jr. 1970. Automated radiometric detection of bacterial growth in blood cultures. J. Lab. & Clin. Med. 75:529–534.
3. DeBlanc, H. J., F. DeLand, and H. N. Wagner, Jr. 1971. Automated radiometric detection of bacteria in 2967 blood cultures. Appl. Microbiol. 22:846–849.
4. Washington II, J. A., and P. K. Yu. 1971. Radiometric method on detection of bacteremia. Appl. Microbiol. 22:100–101.
5. Renner, E. D., L. A. Gatheridge, and J. A. Washington II. 1973. Evaluation of radiometric system for detecting bacteremia. Appl. Microbiol. 26:368–372.

6. Brooks, K. and T. Sodeman. 1974. Rapid detection of bacteremia by a radiometric system. A clinical evaluation. Am. J. Clin. Path. 61:859–866.

7. Smith, A. G., and R. R. Little. 1974. Detection of bacteremia by an automated radiometric method and a tubed broth method. Ann. Clin. Lab. Sc. 4:448–455.

8. Caslow, M., P. D. Ellner, and T. E. Kiehn. 1974. Comparison of the bactec system with blind subculture for the detection of bacteremia. Appl. Microbiol. 28:435–438.

9. Thiemke, W. A., and K. Wicher. 1974. Experiences with a radiometric method for detecting bacteremia in a large county hospital. Ann. Meeting Am. Soc. Microbiol. 112 (Abstr.)

10. Bannatyne, R. M., and N. Harnett. 1974. Radiometric detection of bacteremia in neonates. Appl. Microbiol. 27:1067–1069.

11. Randall, E. L. 1972. Comparison of a radiometric method with conventional cultural methods for detection of bacteremia. Ann. Meeting Am. Soc. Microbiol. 87 (Abstr.)

12. Randall, E. L. 1973. Further studies on a radiometric method for determining bacteremia. Ann. Meeting Am. Soc. Microbiol. 82 (Abstr.)

13. Zwarun, A. A. 1973. Effect of osmotic stabilizers on $^{14}CO_2$ production by bacteria and blood. Appl. Microbiol. 25:589–591.

14. Kulas, C. M., H. B. Short, E. L. Speck, R. F. Betts, and R. G. Robertson. 1974. An evaluation of ^{14}C-labeled osmotically stabilized blood culture media in an automated blood culture system. Ann. Meeting Am. Soc. Microbiol. 112 (Abstr.)

15. Rosner, R. 1974. Comparison of macroscopic, microscopic, and radiometric examinations of clinical blood cultures in hypertonic media. Appl. Microbiol. 28:644–646.

16. DeLand, F. H. 1972. Metabolic inhibition as an index of bacterial susceptibility to drugs. Antimicrob. Agents Chemother. 2:405–412.

17. DeBlanc, H. J., P. Charache, and H. N. Wagner, Jr. 1972. Automatic radiometric measurement of antibiotic effect on bacterial growth. Antimicrob. Agents Chemother. 2:360–366.

18. Previte, J. J. 1972. Radiometric detection of some food-borne bacteria. Appl. Microbiol. 24:535–539.

19. Previte, J. J., R. Wells, and D. B. Rowley. 1974. Radiometric detection of non-fermentors of glucose. Ann. Meeting Am. Soc. Microbiol. 112 (Abstr.)

20. Camargo, E. E., S. M. Larson, B. S. Tepper, P. Charache, and H. N. Wagner, Jr. 1974. Radiometric detection of M. tuberculosis and M. lepraemurium. J. Nucl. Med. 15:481.

21. Larson, S. M., P. Charache, M. Chen, and H. N. Wagner, Jr. 1974. Inhibition of the metabolism of streptococci and Salmonella by specific antisera. Appl. Microbiol. 27:351–355.

22. Keusch, G. T., and S. D. Douglas. 1973. Radiometric screening test for chronic granulomatous disease. J. Nucl. Med. 14:591–594.

23. Larson, S. M., T. Merz, and H. N. Wagner, Jr. 1974. Radiometric screening test of cell-mediated immunity based on phytohemagglutinin (PHA) induced changes in lymphocyte carbohydrate metabolism. J. Nucl. Med. 15:510.

24. Waters, J. R., and A. A. Zwarun. 1973. Results of an automated radiometric sterility test as applied to clinical blood cultures. Develop. Indust. Microbiol. A.I.B.S. 14:80–89.

CHAPTER 14

The Use of Gas Chromatography for the Identification of Microorganisms

Robert J. Mandle and Thomas J. Wade

The process of identification of bacteria and yeasts is essentially based on an examination of their biochemical activity. The use of differential media has been an integral part of the identification of bacteria for almost 100 years.

In 1968, Mitruka and his associates attempted to use the gas chromatograph to identify viruses (1). Previously Moore and his associates at Virginia Polytechnic Institute had used gas chromatography as one parameter in the identification of anaerobic bacteria (2). A search of the literature revealed that the techniques had not only been applied to viruses, but indeed the concept of identification of bacteria by means of gas chromatography was suggested in a paper by Asselineau as early as 1961, in which he suggested that the gas chromatograph might be used in the systematics of bacteria (3). Two years later a similar suggestion was made independently by Abel, de Schmertzing, and Peterson (4). Reiner (5) also published his independent observations on the use of the gas chromatograph to identify microorganisms. Thus, within approximately one decade following the first description of the instrument, its unique attributes were already applied to the problems of bacterial taxonomy.

One of the features of the system which makes it attractive to microbiologists is the very high degree of sensitivity and resolution possessed by the gas liquid chromatograph. It is relatively easy to operate, and relative to most of our modern instrumentation is not an extremely expensive instrument. The approaches which have been applied to the identification of micro-organisms may be broken down into three main groups.

IDENTIFICATION TECHNIQUES FOR BACTERIA AND YEASTS

A. The Detection of Products of Growth in Media

All who have worked with bacteria soon become aware of the fact that there are certain aromatic components elaborated by the growth of bacteria. Many technologists utilize their olfactory senses as an important part of their initial observations of cultures. The gas chromatograph has been used to detect the different components found in the head gases of culture media in which pure cultures of bacteria had been grown (6).

Another variation of this technique has been the one in which components which accrue in the spent media in which bacteria have grown are determined by means of gas-liquid chromatographic procedures. An example of this has been the application of the method of anaerobes by Moore and his co-workers at Virginia Polytechnic Institute (2). This not only revolutionized the approaches to the taxonomy of this difficult group but it also made the gas chromatograph an accepted instrument in the bacteriology laboratory. It facilitated the identification of specific carboxylic acids which were extracted from standard growth media in which the anaerobes were cultivated. A similar approach had been used to extract metabolic products from the broth in which the organisms had grown (7) and to obtain a "signature" from the chromatograph which was suggested to be indicative of the organism.

B. A Different Approach Is That of Examining the Components of the Organism Itself

Reiner (5) used the technique of pyrolysis (exposing the organisms to very high temperatures) to break up the inherent components of the bacterial cells and then to examine these products in the gas chromatograph. The breakdown products resulting from the pyrolysis of the bacterial cells create their own unique "pyrogram" or fingerprint of the bacterial culture. Strains of *Escherichia coli* having different antigenic properties, a *Shigella, Streptococcus pyogenes,* and several mycobacteria provided the pyrograms that might form a new basis for taxonomy. Pyrolysis has similarly been applied to the study of dermatophytes (8). One of the problems of this application is that the pyrolysis technique requires that the cells be dried and usually a known amount placed in the pyrolizer for the gas chromatographic examination so as to help control variability.

Another approach to the problem of preparing cells for examination by gas chromatography is to digest the entire cell by one of a variety of available methods.

A significant change in the way in which the digestates could be made was introduced by McGee (9). He showed that tetramethylammonium hydroxide (TMAH) could be used as the digesting agent to produce usable digestates which did not need to be extracted following removal of the water. Resuspension of the material in alcohol and centrifugation to remove the insoluble material rendered the sample suitable for injection into the chromatograph. This method has been applied to mammalian tissues as well as to a few microorganisms.

C. Detection of In Vivo Grown Microorganisms

The gas chromatograph has been used to detect microorganisms directly in body fluids (10). More recently, the causative agent of a urinary tract infection has been detected by identifying specific amines in the urine obtained from the patient (11). This represents the obvious goal of the application to a rapid diagnostic method.

It is a very time-consuming procedure to identify intestinal anaerobes and we were interested in determining whether it was possible to apply the fingerprint approach suggested in the early work of Reiner (5), McGee (9), and others to this problem. A goal was to determine if an isolate provided a fingerprint which indicated that it was from a novel organism or was one that had previously been identified. I became rather excited about the prospect of this approach and visualized in my naive state that it would be possible very quickly to make a black box, which functioning by a turn-key approach would readily identify the organism.

The techniques of McGee (9) were used first and these were simplified to a one-step digestion of the bacteria. It is these studies on the nonfermenting Gram negative rods which established the reliability and simplicity of the procedure (12).

METHODS

Bacteria to be subjected to examination in the gas chromatograph were grown overnight at 37°C on trypticase soy agar to which 0.2% glucose and 0.2% yeast extract were added (TYG).

A. Preparation of Gas Chromatographic Samples

Cells are prepared for gas chromatographic analysis by one of two methods.

1. Glass Ampule Method Approximately 100 to 800 mm² of bacterial growth is harvested from the growth medium and transferred to a 1-ml glass ampule. The area of growth harvested from each plate is dependent on the amount of growth present and the particular analytical parameters which are to be used and which relate primarily to the total attenuation which is to be applied to the gas chromatographic signal.

The harvesting of cells and their transfer to the glass ampule is accomplished by using an 80-mm^2 long segment of glass capillary which has its terminal portion bent in the form of a 3- by 3-mm glass hook. Bacteria are collected in the open portion of the hook by lightly scraping them off of the agar surface. Care must be taken not to cut into the agar or otherwise pick up extraneous materials. The gas capillary with its occluded cell mass is placed directly into the ampule and the cell mass is not washed. Two drops (approximately 50 microliters) of a saturated methanolic solution of tetramethyl pentahydrate (TMAH) (Southwestern Chemicals Inc., Austin, Texas) is placed into the bottom of the ampule with a Pasteur pipette. The ampule is then sealed under a slight vacuum and heated for 15 min at 100°C. If the sample is not to be analyzed immediately it is stored at −10°C. Routinely, immediately prior to the analysis of each sample, the ampule is opened and the contents transferred to a capped polyethylene microfuge tube (0.4-ml capacity) which then is centrifuged in a Beckman model 152 microfuge for 60 sec in order to sediment any cellular material not solubilized by the sample preparation procedure. If repeat analyses are to be performed on the sample, the capped microfuge tube is stored at −10°C. Long-term storage of samples is done at −60°C.

2. Aluminum Capsule Method *(a) Preparation of the harvesting tool:* The harvesting of organisms for this sampling method is done by using a segment of glass tubing which has its terminal end shaped into a 1- to 2-mm glass sphere. These tools are individually made by heat-drawing the middle portion of the narrow end of a 9-in Pasteur pipette into an 18-in length of very thin glass. This thin glass is broken so that what was formerly the dropping end of the pipette has a 3-in glass segment at one end. A 1- to 2-mm diameter glass sphere is produced at the end of this segment by rapidly melting the glass in a flame.

(b) Preparation of aluminum capsule samples: Routinely, organisms are harvested by collecting an approximately 20 mm^2 area of growth onto the glass sphere. Single colonies of bacteria also are harvested in this manner. The glass sphere, together with its added bacteria, is dipped into an indi-aliquot of 2M methanolic TMAH solution. The sphere, together with its occluded organisms and occluded TMAH solution, is removed from the reagent solution immediately and cut away from the harvesting tool directly into the bottom of a 0.05-ml capacity aluminum capsule. The sphere then is sealed into the capsule by use of a crimping tool designed for this purpose (Perkin-Elmer Corporation). The sealed capsule then is placed into the magazine holder of a Perkin-Elmer AS41 automatic sampling system.

An important point to note here is that the digesting reagent is a saturated methanolic solution of the **TMAH**. This modification of McGee's procedure permits the preparation time to be shortened.

B. Gas Chromatography

The gas chromatographs used in these studies are a Perkin-Elmer model and a Perkin-Elmer model 3920. The former was automated by means of a Perkin-Elmer AS41 automatic sampling system. The columns used are either polyester columns diethylene succinate (DEGS) or high polarity cyanosilicone (SP2300) both from Supelco, Inc., Bellefonte, Pa. The carrier gas is helium and a flame ionization detection system is used. The injector temperature is 320°C, and a temperature program begins at 80°C for 4 min and is increased to 195°C at 8°/min. A final hold time is 20 min.

When an aliquot of the digestate is injected into the gas chromatograph, the high temperature of the injector breaks up the quaternary ammonium salts which are generated during the digestion into their respective fatty acid methyl esters and other components of the bacterial cells. This takes advantage of the large number of unique compounds, including some unique fatty acids, to be found in bacteria and it is the comparison of these which makes the techniques possible.

RESULTS OF STUDIES ON BACTERIA AND FUNGI

The top half of Figure 1 shows a typical chromatogram of *Pseudomonas aeruginosa*. There are many peaks of varying size, having within them different areas. Nearly every sample of bacteria that we examined contained a peak that apparently corresponds with that of methyl palmitate. This became the reference peak which enabled the setting of a peak height and retention time by defining that for methyl palmitate as unity. Thus, it is possible to produce normalized chromatograms, as seen in the lower half of Figure 1, and automatically make allowance for the differences in concentration of cells from sample to sample.

Figure 2 shows the comparison of *P. aeruginosa* and three other *Pseudomonas* species. Over 58 strains of *P. aeruginosa,* and perhaps overall more than 250 strains of nonfermenting organisms, have been examined. In some instances only a few strains and in other instances 15 or 20 strains of species were examined. Looking at these 4, however, you can see that there are distinct differences evidenced in these normalized patterns.

At the same time that we were studying the Pseudomonads, Moss, Samuels, and Weaver at the Center for Disease Control working on the same group, employed analytical techniques to see if there were differences in the

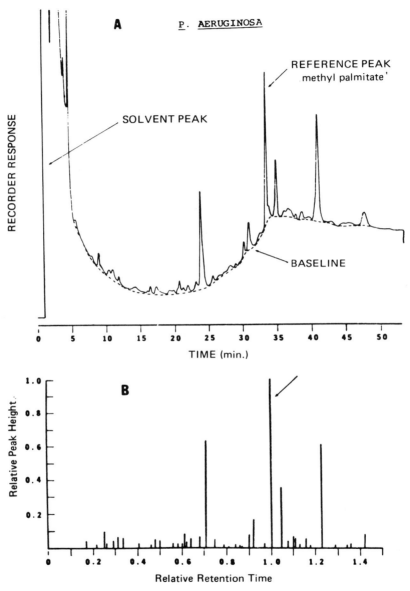

Figure 1. Comparison of the gas chromatograph (*A*) and the normalized profile (*B*) of the chromatographic peaks obtained from a TMAH-digested sample of *P. aeruginosa* strain GC56. (This figure is reproduced with permission of T. J. Wade and R. J. Mandle (12).)

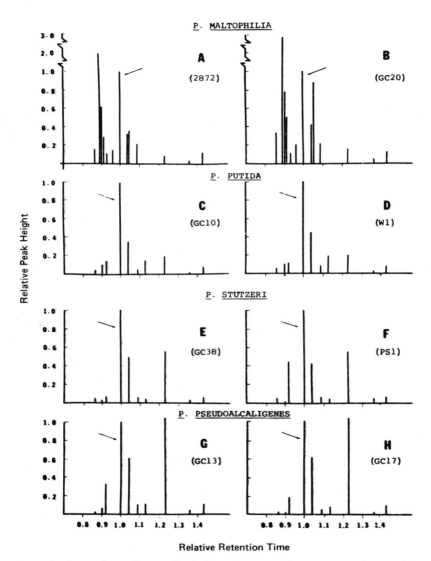

Figure 2. Comparison of normalized chromatograms of two strains of each of four species of *Pseudomonas*.

fatty acid composition of a number of the pseudomonads (13). They suggested such results might correlate with taxonomic differences.

In Figure 2, a comparison is shown of four strains of *Pseudomonas, P. maltophilia, P. putida, P. stutzeri,* and *P. pseudoalcaligenes.* In each instance, two known strains have been compared and there are distinct differences among members of this genus. Therefore, there is the possibility that a very simple digestion system can be used in the preparation of samples for examination in the gas chromatograph. This may not produce a type of digestate suitable for analytical methods, but it is apparent from this slide that it does give the necessary differentiation to allow one to separate members of the genus. This means that this technique has the potential of being utilized in the clinical laboratory as a means of rapid simple identification of microorganisms.

The above chromatograms were obtained on a research chromatograph. As a result of the increased interest in anaerobic bacteria, a simplified version of the gas chromatograph is rapidly becoming a part of the instrumentation in many clinical microbiological laboratories. This less sophisticated instrument does not involve a temperature program. An attempt was made to see if the digestion procedure would be applicable to this isothermal type of gas chromatograph. We found that this methodological approach could be used with a polyester column if a sample is run for a long enough period of time.

The technique has proved to be simple, short, and reproducible because we could identify the nonfermenting Gram negative rods in about 35 min, and it seems to be reliable because, after studying approximately 50 strains of *P. aeruginosa,* the amount of variability has been almost nil.

Major David Ohashi, while working in our laboratory, was able to obtain 10 species of mycobacterium, with at least 3 to 8 strains of each species. Using essentially the same technique as previously described for the pseudomonads, he was able to differentiate the 10 species of mycobacteria. Figure 3 shows a typical chromatogram of *Mycobacterium tuberculosis* and its extremely extended time line. The one shown was run for 2 hr on the gas chromatograph in order to bring out the high molecular weight components which seem to be unique in Mycobacteria. In addition, there is the center portion, which is marked off into three areas. These three areas are very useful for the differentiation of the acid fast bacteria. In all samples of *M. tuberculosis,* there is the late peak seen at the far right-hand end of this chromatograph (Figure 3). This peak has not been found on any of the other strains that have been examined. Before it can be concluded that this is unique to *M. tuberculosis,* it will be necessary to examine many more strains and species of the genus.

Figure 4 shows normalized chromatograms of 10 species of *Mycobacterium.* By observing the magnitude and the presence or absence of given components as indicated by the bars on the normalized chromatogram, it is possible to speciate the members of the genus.

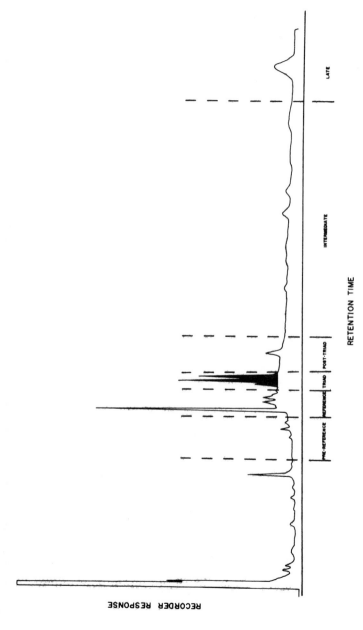

Figure 3. A chromatogram of *Mycobacterium tuberculosis*.

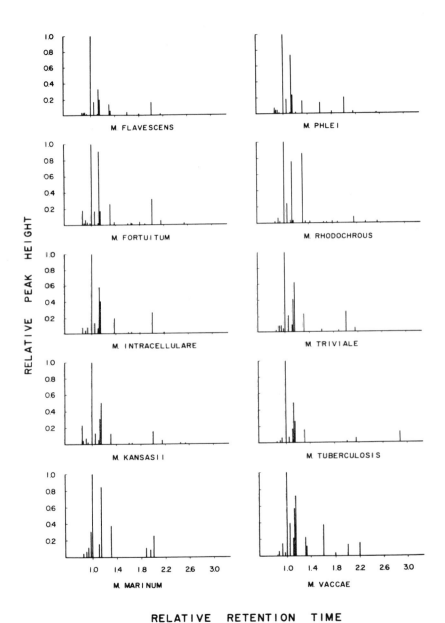

RELATIVE   RETENTION   TIME

Figure 4. Normalized chromatograms of 10 species of *Mycobacterium*.

Preliminary studies have been done on yeasts (Figure 5). These chromatograms suggest that there are indeed generic differences which may permit the separation of these organisms. The data in Figure 5 may tend to support the suggestion of a close taxonomic relationship between *Cryptococcus* and *Rhodotorula*. Limited findings of the possibility of speciation within the genus *Candida* are seen in Figure 6. While only a few strains of some of the yeasts have been studied, it is again highly suggestive that speciation within the genus may be possible.

Since the title of this symposium includes the word "trend," I should like to describe what we hope will be a trend. Automation in microbiology has been very slow in coming. Certainly the progress in automation that has been achieved in the clinical chemistry laboratory is not available in the microbiology laboratory in regard to the identification of microorganisms. It has been mentioned that one idealistic view of the potentials of the gas chromatograph is to consider it as a black box system for use in a clinical microbiology laboratory. We have pursued this idea with the following results.

Being convinced that the technique is reliable, we undertook to improve upon the data handling so that advantage might be taken of some of the ancillary equipment available for the gas chromatograph. One approach to

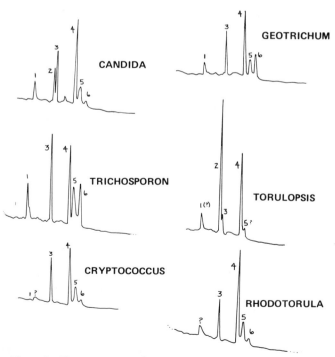

Figure 5. Chromatograms of yeasts representing six different genera.

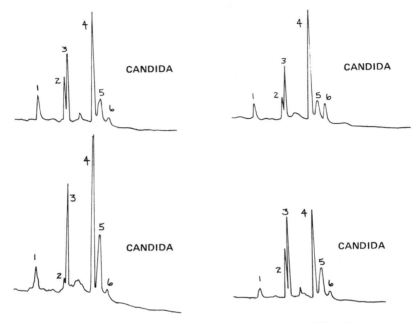

Figure 6. Chromatograms of four different species of *Candida*.

this has been to divide the chromatogram into segments as may be seen in Figure 7. Based on our experience with the pseudomonads, the chromatogram was arbitrarily divided into lettered areas representing those areas wherein major peaks of interest seem most often to occur. A computerized peak detection and integration system received the chromatographic signal and determined the relative retention time versus the relative area for each peak. From these, all of the relative areas can be totalled and a value termed the "sum of the segment relative areas" (SSRA) obtained. Thus, by means of a mini-computer to handle the problem of retention time and area measurement, and a programmable calculator to handle the data produced by the integration system, it is possible to rapidly characterize many more strains of the nonfermenting Gram negative rods. In all, more than 200 strains from collections and clinical isolates were examined with this data processing procedure.

The data obtained from the examination of 58 strains of *Pseudomonas aeruginosa*, 5 of *P. putida*, 4 of *P. stutzeri*, and 6 of *P. pseudoalcaligenes* is seen in Figure 8. The solid black bar indicates the range of SSRA values observed for all of the isolates tested in this particular instance. The arrows indicate the nonoverlapping ranges which are useful for the characterization of the species. This permits a statistical approach to the handling of the information.

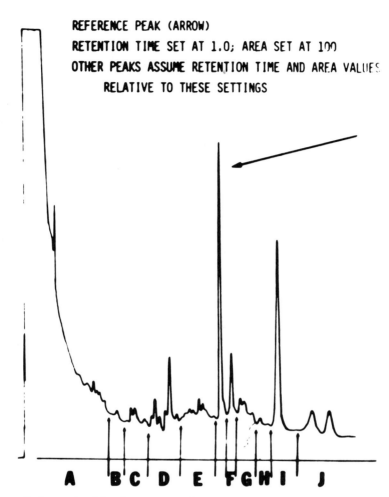

REFERENCE PEAK (ARROW)

RETENTION TIME SET AT 1.0; AREA SET AT 100

OTHER PEAKS ASSUME RETENTION TIME AND AREA VALUES

RELATIVE TO THESE SETTINGS

A   B C   D   E   F G H   I   J

Figure 7. Segments of the chromatogram that are used to compute the segment's sum of the relative areas (SSRA).

The addition of an automatic sample applicator helped to develop this system into something which can have clinical application as a fully automated identification system for bacteria. This was a significant technical advance because it not only allowed for the generation of more data than could easily be handled in a given day, but also, more importantly, it permitted the miniaturization of the sample sizes.

An overall view of the instrumentation that we are currently employing may be seen in Figure 9. At the far left are the controls of the Perkin-Elmer AS41, solvent-free sampling system. The injector itself is positioned on the left side of the model 900 chromatograph. In the upper right is the mini-

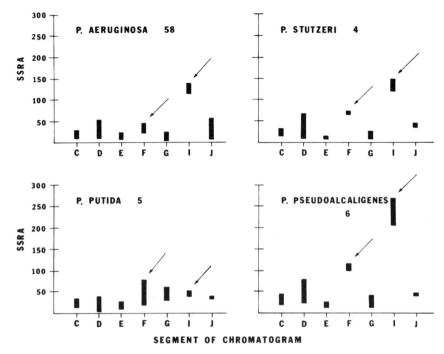

Figure 8. Four species of *Pseudomonas* compared by SSRA values.

computer which receives the output from the gas chromatograph and gives the relative areas and retention values in a printout. This information is then fed into the programmable calculator below it. The wire connection between these two is, at present, the only "missing link" for a completely automated system. We are assured that the necessary wiring can be obtained which will handle the output from the minicomputer directly into the calculator.

Isolated colonies on an agar plate are seen in Figure 10. You will note on the right edge of the plate that there is a Pasteur pipette which has been drawn out so that a small glass sphere is at the terminal end. This sphere is simply touched to an isolated colony and bacteria will adhere to the glass sphere. This then is dipped into methanolic tetramethylammonium hydroxide. The sphere with the bacteria and digesting agent present on it is placed in a small aluminum capsule and the capsule is sealed by means of an instrument which makes a cold weld seal and, thus, takes the place of the heat-sealed ampule in the previous method.

The capsules are loaded in a magazine, and the magazine placed in the feed tray of the automatic sampler. Each sample is then fed sequentially into the gas chromatograph at approximately 35- to 40-min intervals. The capsule is positioned in front of the injection system, punctured so that hot gases

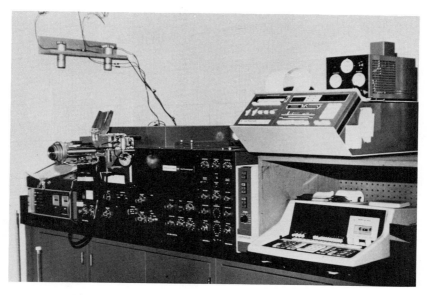

Figure 9. The chromatograph and the auxillary equipment.

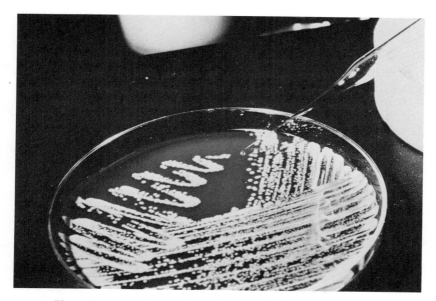

Figure 10. Isolated colonies and the glass probe for sampling a colony.

flow through it, and the digestion of the sample occurs at once. The gases then pass on into the carrier gas that flows into the column. The output from the chromatograph ultimately reaches the programmable calculator where we have previously stored a library of profiles representative of different species of the pseudomonads.

An example of a printout from the calculator is seen in Figure 11. It prints out the number of the strain, the sample, and the chromatogram number. It prints out the data it derives from the sum of the areas within the segments for that particular sample. It "says" at this point: this sample was compared with reference organism number 17 and it has printed out 0000 which means "no match." It furthermore says that the reason there was no match with the stored reference organism was because segment C was too high as indicated by a positive 1, D was too low, F was too low, and G was too high. It also prints out the absolute differences so that one may look at it and decide if the statistics are correct or if a change in the statistics of the system should be considered. In this instance, it said that the strain was not

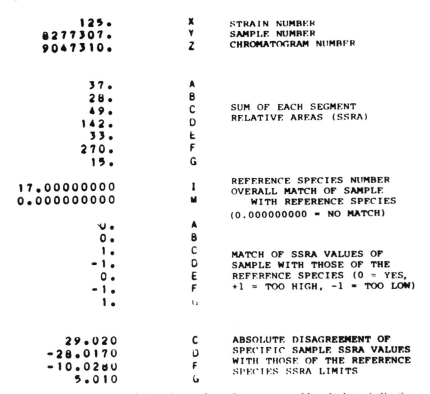

Figure 11. An example of the printout from the programmable calculator indicating a "no match."

similar to the reference strain 17. Had it been close enough, the only part of the above that would have been printed out at this point would have been 17, indicating that the match had been found and it was our reference organism number 17.

SUMMARY

Five years ago, Dr. William B. Cherry of the Center for Disease Control predicted that the gas chromatograph would ultimately become a diagnostic tool in the clinical laboratory. We believe that what I have described today or something very similar to it is a plausible answer to Cherry's vision. The black box is a real possibility now. The gas chromatograph should not only be considered a research instrument, it should be carried one step further than Moore has gone in making it only one parameter of an identification.

If it is possible to name an organism and this information can be related to antibiotic susceptibility patterns, then the name really does become important. We believe that the method described here is very fast and, in reality, the preparation of the sample takes less time than preparing a Gram stain. In addition, the analysis has proved itself to be extremely reliable and, on identical or very similar columns, to be completely reproducible. It is an easy, one-step approach to identification. It is simple because of the innate properties of the digesting reagent. Lastly, we believe that we have shown in our laboratory that it is extremely amenable to automation. Such an automated procedure might give the clinical laboratory a tool which provides at least the accuracy that can now be expected by the use of traditional procedures. More importantly, the answer can be obtained in minutes rather than in hours.

The relatively unsophisticated approach that has been demonstrated as a model now needs the attention of instrument engineers. Computer-controlled gas chromatographs are already available. More specific design of such instrumentation for specific application to microbiological analysis is the next developmental step.

ACKNOWLEDGMENTS

This study was supported in part by project Themis, contract no. N00014-68-0516, Electro-Nucleonics Inc., and the Percival E. and Ethel Brown Foerderer Foundation.

We wish to thank Major David Ohashi for allowing us to cite some of his unpublished work on the identification of the mycobacteria by means of the gas chromatograph.

LITERATURE CITED

1. Mitruka, B. M. 1968. Gas chromatographic detection *in vivo* activity of equine infectious anemia virus. Appl. Microbiol. 16:1093−1094.
2. Moore, W. C. C., E. P. Cato, and L. V. Holdeman. 1966. Fermentation patterns of some Clostridium species. Internat. J. Syst. Bact. 16:383−415.
3. Asselinneau, J. 1961. Sur quelques applications de la chromatographic en phase a l'etude d'acides gras bacteriens. Ann. Inst. Pasteur 100:109−119.
4. Abel, K., H. deSchmertzing, and J. I. Peterson. 1963. Classification of microorganisms by analysis of chemical composition. I. Feasibility of utilizing gas chromatography. J. Bact. 85:1039−1044.
5. Reiner, E. 1965. Identification of bacterial strains by pyrolysis-gas-liquid chromatography. Nature (London) 206:1272−1274.
6. Bassette, R., and T. J. Claydon. 1965. Classification of some bacteria by gas chromatographic analysis of head space vapors from milk cultures. J. Dairy Sci. 48:775 (Abstr.).
7. Henis, Y., J. R. Gould, and M. Alexander. 1966. Detection and identification of bacteria by gas chromatography. Appl. Microbiol. 14:513−524.
8. Carmichael, J. W., A. S. Sekhon, and L. Sigler. 1973. Classification of some dermatophytes by pyrolysis-gas-liquid chromatography. Canad. J. Microbiol. 19:403−407.
9. McGee, J. 1968. Characterization of mammalian tissues and microorganisms by gas-liquid chromatography. J. Gas Chromatogr. 6:48−52.
10. Mitruka, B. M., A. M. Jonas, and M. Alexander. 1970. Rapid detection of bacteremia in mice by gas chromatography. Infect. Immunity 2:474−478.
11. Brooks, J. B., W. B. Cherry, L. Thacker, and C. Alley. 1972. Analysis by gas chromatography of amines produced *in vivo* and *invitro* by *Proteus mirabilis*. Am. Soc. Microbiol. Proc. (Abstr.).
12. Wade, T. J., and R. J. Mandle. 1974. A new gas chromatographic characterization procedure: Preliminary study on *Pseudomonas* species. Appl. Microbiol. 27:303−311.
13. Moss, C. W., S. B. Samuels, and R. E. Weaver. 1972. Cellular fatty acid composition of selected *Pseudomonas* species. Appl. Microbiol. 24:596−598.

CHAPTER 15

The Role of the Computer in Microbiology

Lawrence J. Kunz, James W. Poitras, Jane Kissling,
Bettie A. Mercier, Marion Cameron, Carl Lazarus,
Robert C. Moellering, Jr., and G. Octo Barnett

The use of the computer in microbiology as contrasted with its use in other clinical laboratory disciplines has special significance from two viewpoints. Because of the complexity and the sequential nature of reporting test results in microbiology, a computer-based information system for microbiology is more difficult to design, program, and implement than for other clinical laboratories, such as chemistry and hematology. For example, in clinical chemistry, a laboratory determination will proceed from a null value, such as "results pending," directly to a definitive answer expressed in quantitative terms such as "micrograms per milliliter." Similarly, in hematology, a blood count will proceed from "results pending" in one step to a quantitative result such as "15,000 wbc/cu mm of blood." On the contrary, in microbiology, results are expressed progressively, over a period of days, in increasingly definitive, specific terms, as from "results pending" to "no growth to date" to "moderate numbers of Gram positive cocci" to "moderate Staphylococci" (perhaps with antimicrobial susceptibility tests) to "moderate *Staphylococcus aureus* sensitive or resistant to such and such antimicrobial agents." The requirement for frequent updating of the sequential reports introduces more complex design problems for the microbiology information system than in the chemistry or hematology laboratories.

A computer system in microbiology, however, probably provides more opportunities for usefulness than in other clinical laboratories because of the unique relationship of microbiology to infectious diseases. The advantages of a computer-based information system in microbiology, therefore, include (a) expeditious transmission of results of laboratory determinations to patients' charts; (b) more efficient clerical, fiscal, and administrative housekeeping; (c) effective control of quality and error-avoidance in the performance and reporting of laboratory determinations; and (d) promotion of research relating to basic microbiological procedures and to diagnostic, therapeutic, and epidemiological aspects of infectious diseases.

Normally one would expect that the primary reason to develop a computer system for a laboratory service might be related to the transmission of the results of laboratory determinations from the technologist's bench to the patient's record and that any other benefits might be considered to be secondary gains. In practice, however, one or the other of the so-called secondary gains has more often than not been the primary objective of the introduction of the computer into the clinical laboratory.

Nevertheless, it is usually impossible and nonproductive, as in every aspect of health care, to draw sharp lines between patient care, teaching (or learning), and clinical research. And so it is with a computer-based system in microbiology where concepts such as cost-effectiveness in medical care can only hazily be computed because one patient's "research" leads to another patient's "direct medical care."

This portrayal of the role of the computer in microbiology is presented here using a description of the computer system of the bacteriology laboratory of the Massachusetts General Hospital as the format. This description of the system includes an attempt to elucidate the principles that guided us in the choice of modes, devices, and alternative methods to achieve proposed objectives. It represents one set of points of view in design, and this guiding philosophy will be exemplified and rationalized in the presentation. It is recognized, however, that certain benefits and advantages may be derived from other choices.

Two principles were continuously invoked for guidance when selection between alternate modes, methods, techniques, or choices of any kind had to be made: (a) that a computer system was being adapted to serve the laboratory, its personnel, and our patients and not vice versa; and (b) that avoidance of error and assurance of quality were more important than economy, ease of programming, and similar considerations.

The system was designed and implemented over a number of years through the collaboration of many members of the Francis Blake Bacteriology Laboratories and the Laboratory of Computer Science (LCS) of the Massachusetts General Hospital. The system is still evolving.

MATERIALS AND METHODS

A. Computer, Terminals, and Language

The system runs on a Digital Equipment Corporation PDP 9 or 15 computer with 32K of 18 bit word core, 3 million characters of fixed head disc storage and 24 million characters of moveable head disc storage. The LCS maintains, operates, and programs the computer which is currently dedicated to chemistry and bacteriology laboratory applications. All of the application programs are written in MUMPS (MGH Utility Multi-Programming System) which is an interpretive time-sharing system (1).

Terminals are located in the bacteriology laboratory and are connected directly to the computer via hardwired telephone lines. These terminals, maintained by the LCS, are operated by members of the bacteriology laboratory and consist of teletypes, Infoton CRT (cathode ray tube) terminals, and a Millipore Electronic Zone Analyzer (EZA), maintained by Millipore Corporation, Bedford, Massachusetts for antibiotic susceptibility determinations (2). Reports are printed in the laboratory on an A. B. Dick line-printer.

B. Input Modes

Of the several different modes of entering information into the computer—marked or punched cards and card-readers, numeric codes, coded individual keys on a templated keyboard, etc.—we have chosen to use mnemonic word codes plus the added capability to use free text. This choice was made because we considered it to be less error-prone than the other modalities especially because, with an on-line system, errors in entry or discrepancies between items of data could be detected and easily corrected at the time of entry since source documents were immediately at hand.

As a consequence, code words are used for description of specimens—SP for sputum, CVS for clean voided specimen of urine, LK for left kidney urine, RU for right ureter urine, etc. Incorrect words resulting from errors in typing are not recognized by the computer and are rejected. Entry of results of cultures are similarly made in the form of code words; EC expands to *Escherichia coli*, AERUG expands to *Pseudomonas aeruginosa*, AROG to *Enterobacter aerogenes*, etc. We feel that depressing these few keys per organism with immediate display of input on the CRT is a little more costly of time and effort than manipulating marked spaces on cards; this marginal increase in effort is justified by the benefits of practically simultaneous observation of entered data.

Verification of codes provides for establishment of defined files of storage in the computer and, therefore, for subsequent economical retrieval of data for examination and statistical analysis for purposes of quality control, patient care, research, and fiscal and clerical administrative housekeeping. The capability of utilizing free text for pertinent comments and for elaboration or qualification of laboratory results is a decided advantage. Code words have been established for certain frequently used comments that are convenient to employ, such as: MIXED, mixed bacterial colonies; ? contaminated specimen; or SEC, see earlier culture for sensitivities.

C. Entering Results into the Computer

Results of cultures are entered into the appropriate, previously established specimen files in several ways as will be described presently. When a specimen is received in the laboratory, it is assigned a four-digit number; this specimen number and other identifying characteristics of the specimen are logged into the computer to establish a file. The computer automatically appends as check digits to the specimen number the last two digits of the patient's hospital unit number. This addition reduces by 99% the possibility of gaining access to the wrong specimen file in the computer due to transposition of digits or by other errors in transcribing specimen numbers. An example of the format used in logging in is presented in Figure 1. In this figure, the characters that are manually typed for entry into the computer are underlined; all other characters are automatically typed under direction of the computer, i.e., specimen number, patient's name and location, and the queries UN ("What is the unit number of the patient?") and T ("What test is requisitioned?").

```
02/17   1945  UNUSED     SN:  1945
      INITIALS:  F
      1945
UN  ........     ...   FW
T   SP,C,
    1946
UN  ........     ........   WH6
T   U,C,
    1947
UN  ........     ........   RF3
T   FL-CSF,CS,
    1948
UN  ........     ........   RF5
T   W-SCALP,C,
```

Figure 1. Portion of actual hard copy of logging in specimens. Manually typed material has been underlined to differentiate it from computer-generated typing. Patients' unit numbers and names have been partially obliterated to maintain confidentiality. Explanatory notes: 1945, 1946, etc., specimen numbers; UN, unit number; T, test; 7 digit numbers, patients numbers; EW, WH6, etc., patient care areas.

As soon as a specimen is logged into the computer, the status of the specimen is considered as "pending"; it is changed by entering, subsequently, preliminary or definitive results.

Results are entered as described below; each clinical report supercedes the previous report or status of the specimen; only the latest status is reported because earlier results are ablated whenever updated results are entered into the computer. In general, results are entered as follows:

1. *Smears* of specimens, after being stained and examined, are described in free text. Smears of cultures (e.g., blood cultures) are usually reported in abbreviated form in code words which are translated into full text on printing. Thus, "G+CCH" expands to "Gram positive cocci in chains" on the printed report.

2. *Blood and urine cultures* are automatically changed from status "pending" to, respectively, "negative to date" and "no significant growth" at midnight of the day of planting. Printouts of results are not made on the next day until the positive blood and urine cultures are appropriately resulted in the computer. By this programming device, about one-half of our total volume of work is reported almost automatically since urines constitute about one-third of our volume and blood specimens one-sixth. Positive blood cultures are entered into the computer as Gram stain readings of the broth culture. "Positive" urines are those which are judged to have amounts of colonies empirically correlated with 10^5 or more bacteria/ml of urine; they are entered into the computer under a special program for "positive urine cultures" by typing in only the specimen numbers of the positive cultures.

3. *Preliminary results of other cultures* are entered by specimen number with code words read from copies of original multi-part requisitions submitted by the technologists who have examined the cultures; they are prepared in handwriting, usually in the appropriate code language.

4. *Antibiotic susceptibility test results* are entered into the specimen files directly from the electronic zone analyzer (EZA) whose mini-computer is interfaced with the main laboratory computer. Again, access to the appropriate files is achieved through the specimen number.

5. *Final results* are entered by code words from the original work card, prepared, and completed by the technologists examining the culture.

Entries are usually made in a dialogue form as illustrated in Figure 2. Again, economy of effort (relatively few keyboard characters per unit of information) and on-line capability to detect and correct errors recommended this general approach to entering information over other methods, such as through the medium of punched or mark-sense cards that are machine read or entered into the computer at locations distant from the original source documents.

Although two data-input operators are usually employed for entering results and answering telephone inquiries, a single person can handle the job

```
UN/SN  6571-74        ...........

02/26  11      SN: 6571
    C
ORG/CH: 1844522  FC  CHECK  VERY  RARE  CODE:  Y   AMT:  F   CM/S:

ORG: 5044562  FC    AMT:  V   CM/S :

ORG: FINAL


UN/SN  6690-37        ...........

02/26  CVS        SN:  6690
F   STAPH
ORG/CH:  EPID   AMT:  F   CY/S :
V   G-F
ORG/CH:  5044572  FC    AMT:  F   CM/S :

ORG: FINAL.
```

Figure 2. Example of dialogue format for entering final culture results into computer. Material entered manually (usually not via teletype) has been underlined to differentiate it from computer-generated printout (usually displayed on CRT). Underlined blank spaces signify that an escape key had been depressed to verify and enter preceding typed material or to escape to next computer-generated word.

on a given day, but not without a good deal of concentrated effort. Our current work load amounts to about 1,200 to 1,500 results/day since almost all cultures (600 to 700/day) are reported preliminarily at least once. Since this is an on-line system, inquiries for information can be made throughout the day with access to the computer file either by patient's name or unit number or by specimen number. Information is available in the files for up to 2 months for immediate response to inquiries.

RESULTS

A. Reporting of Clinical Bacteriology Laboratory Test Results

The primary objective at the time of installing the computer system in the MGH Bacteriology Laboratory was to expedite the transmission of clinically relevant information between the laboratory and the patients' charts. An illustration of the manner in which laboratory results are printed for insertion into patients' records is provided in Figure 3, which is a reproduction of an actual cumulative report of bacteriological laboratory data issued on the date specified for a given patient. Similar superceding reports are issued once daily in the late afternoon whenever new information warrants an updated report. (An additional noontime report was discontinued in May 1974 after it was generally considered to be unnecessary and seldom referred to.) A permanent

```
09/04/74  MGH                   ᵀᵁᴿᵀᴵᴴᴬᴿᴷ    BF3    ᴵᵁᵁ ᵁᴸ +ᵁ


.--- URINE

08/30 URINE    SN:7345
#### FINAL REPORT:   NO GROWTH

08/31 URINE    SN:7560
#### FINAL REPORT:   NO GROWTH


--- SPUTUM

08/30 SPUTUM   SN:7171
#### FINAL REPORT:
         SMEAR..MODERATE GRAM POSITIVE COCCI IN CLUSTERS  FEW GRAM
                ..POSITIVE RODS. FEW POLYS, ABUNDANT CELL FRAGMENTS
                ..RARE EPITHELIAL CELLS
         CULTURE:
         ABUNDANT STAPH AUREUS
              PEN R    METH S    ERYTH S    CEPH S    TETRA S
         CHLOR S
         SCANT NORMAL FLORA PRESENT

08/31 SPUTUM   SN:7587
         ABUNDANT STAPH AUREUS
         ? ABUNDANT PNEUMOCOCCI
         NORMAL FLORA PRESENT

08/31 SPUTUM   SN:7623
#### FINAL REPORT:
         ABUNDANT STAPH AUREUS
         SEE EARLIER CULTURE FOR SENSITIVITIES
         ABUNDANT PNEUMOCOCCI
         SCANT NORMAL FLORA PRESENT

09/03 SPUTUM   SN:8478
         ABUNDANT GRAM NEG ROD #1
         ABUNDANT ENTERIC GRAM NEG RODS #2

09/04 SPUTUM   SN:8976
         SMEAR..ABUNDANT GRAM POSITIVE AND GRAM NEGATIVE ORGANISMS OF
                ..MIXED MORPHOLOGY WITH GRAM POSITIVE COCCI IN PAIRS
                ..PREDOMINATING  ABUNDANT POLYS AND CELL FRAGMENTS  RARE
                ..EPITHELIAL CELLS
         CULTURE: PEND


--- BLOOD

08/30 BLOOD-   SN:7323    NEG TO DATE

08/30 BLOOD-   SN:7324    NEG TO DATE
```

Figure 3. Reproduction of an actual report of bacteriology laboratory results printed for insertion in a patient's hospital record. Part of the patient's name and unit number have been obliterated to preserve confidentiality.

summary report, not replaceable, is issued on the last day of the week. Finalized cultures are then removed from the files and a new series of successive cumulative reports are issued daily, when indicated, starting on Sunday.

It will be noted that the format of the report permits the display of results of numerous tests on a single page in a space-saving matrix. All cultures from a given specimen type or body site (urine, blood, etc.) are grouped together in chronological order; results are preliminary unless specified as final. This format, it is believed, saves physical spaces in the patient's record and is time-saving for the physician because all reports of similar determinations are available in juxtaposition for comparative study or analysis.

On the reverse side of the report form are listed notes pertaining to routine procedures and to terms, abbreviations, and explanations of phrases used in formulating reports. For example, considerable attention is given to explanations of which organisms or groups of organisms are sought in cultures of various types of specimens, which organisms are considered to be indigenous to various body sites and are not isolated or reported, and the conditions under which cultures for certain types or classes of bacteria must be specifically requested.

B. Spinoffs

Secondary gains (as opposed to the primary objective) made available through the introduction of computer technology in the bacteriology laboratory are still being exploited, achieved, and anticipated. Easily perceivable and immediately achievable spinoffs were programmed and realized at the inception of our system. Others were acquired later or are yet to be attained. These secondary gains from acquisition of a computer-based information system in microbiology, as perceived in the bacteriology laboratory of the Massachusetts General Hospital, will be briefly described in the following sections. Certain of these are the result of programmed searches of computer files for desired information. These searches are conducted at night and the results are printed out each morning. Other printouts are the result of monthly tabulations of data, still others are retrievals of blocks of data analyzed semiannually, annually, or at other intervals. It will be obvious, in most of the following descriptions, whether the data resulted from a programmed "end of day" search or after a specific monthly or otherwise periodic tabulation.

1. Work cards on which technologists record observations, test set-ups, results of tests, etc. are printed automatically for each specimen immediately after "logging in." The pertinent information on each work card includes name, hospital number and location of patient, specimen number (with the two added "safety digits"), type of specimen, name of physician, and types of media used in original culture (for ease of technologists in recording results). The type of work card to be printed (i.e., for urine culture, blood culture, etc.) is determined by the code words used when logging in the respective specimen types.

2. An alphabetical list by line of all patients from whom specimens have been received, giving name, unit number, location, specimen number, and types of specimen.

3. A numerical listing (accession list) of specimens by line, essentially as in 2 above.

4. A list of patients who have tests or cultures signifying diseases reportable by law to the state or local public health department. (These patients are not reported by the laboratory; line listings are forwarded to the hospital administration for action deemed appropriate.)

5. A list of specimens in the laboratory for 48 hr without having had a preliminary report issued. Since the laboratory work-load is divided more or less equally into four sections alphabetically by patient's name, this list is printed out in four parts, one for each section.

6. Twice weekly listing of cultures not finalized within an arbitrarily specified period of time. A special listing for fungus cultures, with a longer tolerance time, is issued separately.

7. Other housekeeping lists and caveats, such as patients with question of two unit numbers, and lists of mycobacterial and mycological specimens (not reported by computer because of incubation periods so much longer than routine cultures) which require subsidiary sub-sets of specimen numbers and handling outside the computer system.

8. Tapes containing logging in data which are forwarded to the accounting department of the hospital for purposes of charging, billing, and collecting laboratory fees.

9. Ad hoc lists of special searches for unusual organisms, organisms of special interest because of in-house, local, regional, or national interest, etc. Searches such as these can be instituted with little prior notice (hours) and implemented on the same day for purposes of searching patient-specimen-culture-organism files for data of epidemiological, nosocomial, or laboratory interest.

10. Listing of patients with blood cultures positive for new organisms (Figure 4). In context with each organism represented on the list are data showing the number of patients with blood cultures positive for the same organism during the previous quarter of the year, during the present quarter to date, and during the present month to date. This permits epidemiological evaluation of current positive blood cultures in respect to normal expectancy based on previous and current experience.

11. Monthly, a list of numbers of organisms isolated, according to source (urinary tract, respiratory tract, blood, and other sources).

12. Histograms of sizes of zones of inhibition versus numbers of strains for each antibiotic and for each principal organism isolated are printed at the end of every month. These are modeled after the computer generated plots of O'Brien, Kent, and Medeiros (3) and are illustrated in Figure 5.

13. Also printed monthly are tabulations of percentages of each major organism that was found in antibiotic susceptibility tests to be sensitive to the various antibiotics tested. These are compared with the previous one-half year's experience and are broken down by sources of specimens, by certain

```
STAPH AUREUS
( 001 THIS MONTH,  016 THIS QUARTER,  035 LAST QUARTER)
GRAHER, HOONIHA          102-03-40  BM5    3584    09/23/74
```

```
STAPH EPIDERMIDIS
( 002 THIS MONTH,  041 THIS QUARTER,  093 LAST QUARTER)
DI ,NJ, JHLILH           104 ., 01  MREC   4016    03/23/74
DUBOIS, LILLIAN  I        001-05-10  WB12   6832    08/29/74
```

```
STREPTOCOCCI PROBABLY ENTEROCOCCI
( 001 THIS MONTH,  010 THIS QUARTER,  014 LAST QUARTER)
FLABODY, HELKLD          000 11-00   PH6    7366    08/30/74
```

Figure 4. Portion of report of positive blood cultures printed on 9/2/74 for epidemiological analysis.

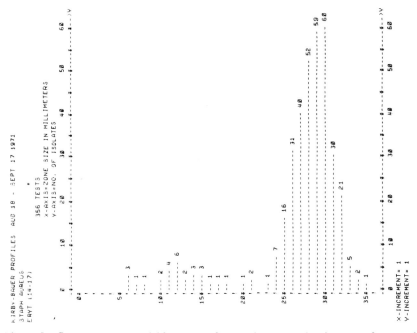

Figure 5. Computer-generated histogram of zone sizes occurring in tests of susceptibility of 356 strains of *Staphylococcus aureus* to erythromycin.

hospital services, and according to whether the cultures were derived from inpatients or outpatients. In addition, percentages are listed both for total isolates and for totals corrected for replicate isolates with the same suceptibility pattern from the same patient, i.e., for unique isolates.

14. Monthly tallies of numbers of specimens according to type (blood, urine, sputum, etc.). The monthly data are derived from daily cumulative totals that are printed out each morning showing numbers of specimens received that day compared to the totals for the month to date.

15. Numbers of biotypes by profile number (Analytab Products, Inc.) of each biotypable Gram negative organism with the percentages of the total number of the species represented by each biotype. These data are collected and analyzed for epidemiological implications and for quality control of laboratory performance.

16. Several of the collections of data made at monthly intervals are tallied for periods of 6 months, 1 year, and longer, for statistical analysis and observation, and for providing bases for comparison with other blocks of data. Figure 6, depicting distributions of sizes of zones of inhibition for tobramycin and gentamicin against some 10,000 strains of *E. coli*, suggests the tremendous amount of computations saved by processing information such as this by computer.

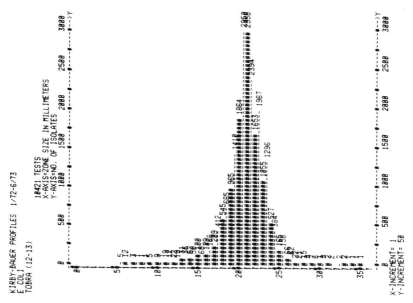

Figure 6. Comparison of distribution of zone sizes for gentamicin (*vertical dashes*) and tobramycin (*cross-hatched figures*) against *Escherichia coli*. Computer-generated plots for organisms tested during an 18-month period are superimposed, slightly out of register.

Analysis of this type of data has also provided us with a basis for designing programs for detection and correction of real or potential discrepancies between antibiotic susceptibility patterns and identification of microorganisms. There are now some 20 sets of criteria in the computer for challenging possible mistesting of microorganisms. Such discrepancies are searched for nightly and printed out the next morning in a format that also suggests steps to be taken to test and, if necessary, confirm or change the apparently unsatisfactory data. This is not only an automated quality control procedure but also an effective device for teaching technologists meaningful laboratory procedures. An example of such a work pattern is illustrated in Figure 7.

SUMMARY AND CONCLUSIONS

Certain potential applications of a computer-based system not included in the system described above are (a) access to information in the computer via remote terminals (e.g., in patient care areas) either by direct inquiry through keyboard with response by CRT or teletype, or by direct printout of patients' reports in patient care areas under either local or central control; or (b) computer-assisted identification of microorganisms by comparison in the computer of test results of unknown strains with biochemical matrices in storage or on file. Although this is obviously an interesting and intellectually challenging use of the computer, it has not seemed to us to be an immediately attractive one in comparison with other priorities.

Another lesser exploited potential for the computer has been its role in detection and prediction of nosocomial epidemics. Although information of epidemiological interest has been made available by the computer on a regular basis, the full potential of the computer system for epidemiological purposes has not as yet been realized. It must be emphasized that we are not concerned

```
3D3-38-24   UILLSSNDJ WILLS.... ..   7451-24   MISC-  (ENTEROCOCCI--METH)

PROBLEM:  METHICILLIN SENSITIVE ENTEROCOCCI

    1. REPEAT SENSI                 STILL 14 OR MORE?   YES....NO....
       ZONE SIZE....

    2. IF 'YES' SET UP THE FOLLOWING:
          ARGININE                           POS....NEG....
          SUCROSE AGAR (GUMDROP COLONIES)    POS....NEG....
          STARCH HYDROLYSIS                  POS....NEG....

    3. IS ORGANISM S. BOVIS?               YES....NO....

    4. IF NOT BOVIS REFER FOR GROUPING     GROUP.........
```

Figure 7. Example of computer-generated report of one type of apparent discrepancy between antibiotic susceptibility and identification of an organism. Procedure to be followed for resolving the apparent conflict is included in the printout.

with utilization of the computer to perform calculations of statistics collected by infection control officers or epidemiologists in the course of making rounds on patients with infections. Rather we should like the computer to analyze information available to it automatically from already existing data banks and, as an occasional consequence, to give early warning of an incipient or on-going epidemic. Such data banks may be accumulated from patient information collected in the admitting office, culture results including biotype and susceptibility patterns, the normal expectancy of types of organisms isolated in given patient areas or from certain anatomic sites, etc. The accumulation of the data already available to the computer, we think, should provide sufficient information so that properly specified manipulation of the data might result in early detection of possible epidemics (i.e., higher than expected incidence of disease).

The introduction of a computer system in the bacteriology laboratory of the Massachusetts General Hospital has been eminently successful in achieving the objectives for which it was designed, objectives that clearly do not include all of the capabilities of the computer in medical microbiology. The applications of the system have not been exhausted and we are particularly interested in further exploiting the system for epidemiological purposes.

LITERATURE CITED

1. Barnett, G. O. 1974. The modular hospital information system. *In* B. Waxman and R. W. Stacy (eds.), Computers in Biomedical Research. Vol. 4, pp. 243—266. Academic Press, Inc., New York.
2. Moellering, Jr., R. C., B. A. Mercier, L. J. Kunz, and J. W. Poitras. 1972. Evaluation of a computer-associated electronic zone analyzer in single-disc antimicrobial susceptibility testing. Antimicrob. Agents Chemother. 2: 95—102.
3. O'Brien, T. F., R. L. Kent, and A. A. Medeiros. 1969. Computer-generated plots of results of antimicrobial-susceptibility tests. J. A. M. A. 210:84—92.

Summary of the Conference

Vern Pidcoe

Changes and innovations in clinical microbiology present a multiplicity of facets and subjects from government regulation through convenience package kits to various stages of mechanization, automation, and computerization. As a result, the program committee of this symposium recognized the impossibility of covering all aspects within the 2 days available. Therefore some major areas of the subject were arbitrarily selected and the speakers were charged with the responsibility of "capsulating" their topics into summary form.

The prime objective of this symposium has been to provide some information which will be useful in planning and in making decisions for progressive laboratory development. As a result, some specific information, examples and an overview are provided to update the audience on many of the regulatory and technical facets of clinical microbiology and immunology.

In his keynote address, Dr. Sherris acknowledged the many changes in the past decade which bear upon the clinical laboratory and seemed to sound a note of impatience that we are still moving too slowly toward automation and mechanization in microbiology. He predicted the adoption of more sophisticated and totally new approaches in clinical microbiology and immunology. Most important, perhaps, he reminded us that the ultimate purpose of all these past, present, and future changes is "to develop the means of providing the optimal data required for patient care as reliably and econom-

195

ically possible and as rapidly as can be achieved in cases of clinical urgency." He cautioned that automatically produced "redundant data may obscure rather than illuminate, and that the seeking of levels of precision which are clinically irrelevant may enhance cost without value to the patient or the science." Further, the application of judgment based on knowledge and experience will never be replaced by automation, but rather automation will simply extend the capability of the clinical microbiologist. He pointed to the need for "greater attention to the quality of specimens and to using all available procedures to assess the pathogenic role of organisms in mixed cultures." In short, he successfully placed the subject of the symposium into appropriate perspective.

Mr. Blatt reviewed the federal program calling for a uniform labeling format for all in vitro diagnostic products and for the establishment of product class standards for groups of in vitro diagnostic products. The only proposed standard to date is for the detection and measurement of glucose. However, he announced that the next three calls for data (nontreponemal tests for syphilis, rabies, and rubella) based on the needs of the profession and patients, are products used in the microbiological sector. Most important was his plea for response to FDA activities from professional groups and stressed the desire of FDA to cooperate with professionals and manufacturers.

Dr. Stickney reviewed the CLIA which addresses itself to personnel, quality control, facilities and equipment, and proficiency testing. He indicated that HEW will continue to increase its regulation of clinical laboratory practice in order to achieve "one set of standards uniformally applied."

The important role of one state by way of example in the training and education of laboratorians at all levels was reviewed by Dr. Hausler. He emphasized the need for state health laboratories to participate in all phases of development and improvement of the skills needed in the health laboratory setting. He indicated some resistance to federal activities in the laboratory area and proposed a compromise in which uniform regulations are administered by the state.

In Section II, Dr. Martin presented an overview of the basic trends in design for the rapid detection of bacteria or their products. He envisions a mild revolution in the microbiology laboratory, although not of the magnitude which transformed methodology in clinical chemistry and hematology. He voiced a note of caution that "Impressive as these detection systems appear to be for the most part, much more investigative work and many more evaluations will be needed to prove their worth in the laboratory on a day-to-day basis." He also pointed out that most microbiology laboratories are not in a position to undertake programs to evaluate such systems.

It was stressed by Dr. Isenberg that all rapid identification systems for Enterobacteriacae are still based upon the "ancient biochemical modalities of taxonomy." He considers all systems to be intermediate in the search for rapid identification procedures and called for permitting modern technology to bear on the problem.

Dr. Cherry expressed some disappointment in the extent to which IF has become a routine procedure in the laboratory. However, he did indicate that IF for *C. diphtheriae* and for *Neisseria gonorrhoeae* was unacceptable as a diagnostic tool at this time. He stressed the potential usefulness of IF for enteropathogenic *Escherichia coli* in hospital laboratories and he expressed his feeling that undo criticism has been heaped upon the FTA-ABS test. It should not be used for screening, and "false" positives may be declared without solid justification.

The routine susceptibility testing of anaerobes was discouraged by Mrs. Nygaard. She also stressed that oxygen must be completely excluded if anaerobes are to be isolated successfully. To this end, the careful selection of equipment and methods for anaerobic isolation must be selected with great care.

Recent progress in immunological diagnosis of bacterial and fungal diseases has been limited to the fungal and syphilitic diseases. However, Dr. Palmer noted that a need exists for more commercially available fungal reagents. He also emphasized that the typhoid H and O agglutination tests should be abandoned in favor of isolation of the organism.

Large hospital laboratories should have virus diagnostic laboratories, at least for primary isolation with the back-up of referral laboratories for identification. Dr. Plotkin further stressed the potential of the indirect IF method for the diagnosis of certain viral diseases and toxoplasmosis. He anticipated the commercial availability of many of the necessary IF reagents within the next 5 years.

EBV-IgM antibody tests can be particularly useful in the diagnosis of selected borderline cases of infectious mononucleosis, but tests are available in relatively few laboratories. Dr. Joncas emphasized that most cases of mononucleosis are identified by the Paul Bunnell-Davidsohn test, particularly if carried out with horse cells. This still seems to be the most reliable procedure.

Dr. Rose noted that large numbers of autoimmune tests are now being done in most laboratories and cited those for rheumatoid factor and anti-nuclear antibody as examples. He predicted that even more tests for autoimmune antibody should be anticipated and that these could be carried out in any normally well-equipped clinical laboratory. However, he cautioned that tests must be adjusted to clinical significance. Finally, he echoed Dr. Plotkin in stressing the potential usefulness of the indirect IF test methodology.

The broad potential use of RIA as applied to microbiology was presented by Dr. Fleisher. He cited RIA and competitive protein binding as techniques now in use to recognize some bacterial antigens and to identify certain microorganisms. He pointed out that because the techniques are rapid, sensitive to detection of picograms of antigen, and relatively inexpensive, the concept of their routine use is very attractive. However, there are drawbacks which will require cooperative research and development between the microbiologist and the biochemist. He predicted that "Radioimmunoassay applied to microbiology will eliminate costly unnecessary work as well as provide information of greater clinical relevance."

The BACTEC system is an example of the radiometric technique for the early detection of bacterial growth. Dr. Randall described the technique as faster than traditional procedures and capable of detecting more positive blood cultures with a saving of personnel time. It appears to be a front runner in revolutionizing the break with the traditional 18- to 24-hr time interval which has dominated the clinical microbiology laboratory for most of our life time.

"Basic gas chromatograph has won acceptance in the clinical laboratory," according to Dr. Mandle. He described a nearly automated technique capable of identifying some microorganisms in less than 1 hr. The technique which he described uses a simple digestate rather than pyrolysis which requires dried organisms in measured quantities. The method has been successful in identifying and characterizing strains of many *Pseudomonas* species, mycobacteria, and certain yeasts.

Dr. Kunz discussed the present availability of computers for assistance in identifying members of the Enterobacteriaceae when either of two kit systems are used by the clinical laboratory. Furthermore, he presented the use of the computer in the microbiology laboratory of the Massachusetts General Hospital, where it is used from logging in the specimen to printing the test results on the patient's chart. The most automated of its uses involves the incorporation of a television zone reader for susceptibility testing coupled directly to the computer. Dr. Kunz cited numerous spin-off advantages of the computerized system, e.g., billing, determining total numbers in a selected category, checking on whether a report has gone out, selecting diseases reportable to the health department, and epidemiological surveillance.

It seems clear that we are in an era of transition from traditional practices in clinical microbiology and immunology into a revolution of new technological advances and concepts. The traditionalists among us will tend to resist these changes while the more progressive and impatient among us will break completely with tradition and rush to embrace all things new. It behooves us to strike the balance between these two extremes. We must acknowledge that clinical microbiology and immunology have lagged behind in providing rapid, clinically relevant data. We must move quickly, but not hastily, to correct this problem. We must recognize also that the innovations are just beginning! Select carefully from that which is currently available to meet the need, but look to the future for continued changes in concepts and improvements in technology and, again, select carefully from them. We have had a good look at what is and what is developing. Now, let us apply it for the good of the patient and science.

Index

Analylab Products, Inc. (API) system, 45–46
Aspergillosis, 95
Autoantibodies in human diseases, 129
Autoimmune diseases, laboratory diagnosis, 127–141

Bacteremia, 153–157
Bacteria
  anaerobic
    antibiotic susceptibility testing, 78–79
    collection and transportation, 67–68
    isolation methods, 68–74
    primary handling and biochemical testing, 75–78
    systems for isolation and identification of, 67–82
  chromatographic identification techniques, 164–165
  enteric, 88
  in food, 158
  identification, 158–159
  immunofluorescence tests for, 51–65
  immunological diagnosis of diseases from, 87–98
  rapid detection in clinical specimens, 29–39
  results of chromatographic studies, 167–179
  serology, 88–93
Bacteriology
  clinical and public health application of direct IF tests, 61

applications of indirect IF tests, 52–61
  computerized reporting of clinical laboratory test results, 186–188
  needs and future directions of IF testing, 61–62
Bacteriuria, mini-culture methods for detection of, 36–37
Blastomycosis, 96
Blood, autoimmune diseases, 136–137
Brucella, 88–90

Candidiasis, 96
Center for Disease Control, role in technology transfer, 11–14
Chromatography
  gas, preparation of samples, 165–167
  gas-liquid, 32–34
  identification of microorganisms by, 163–180
  results of studies on bacteria and fungi, 167–179
Clinical Laboratory Improvement Act, 11–14
Coccidioidomycosis, 96
Computer
  entering results into, 184–186
  input modes, 183
  in microbiology, 181–193
  spinoffs, 188–192
  terminals and language, 183
Connective tissue, autoimmune diseases, 137–138
Cryptococcosis, 96–97
Cytomegalovirus, 100–101

Detection, rapid, of bacteria in
    clinical specimens, 29–39
Diagnosis
    immunological, of bacterial and
        fungal diseases, 87–98
    laboratory
        of autoimmune diseases,
            127–141
        of infectious mononucleosis,
            105–125
    rapid, of viral infections, 99–104
Diagnostic products, in vitro, FDA
    regulation of, 7–10
Diseases
    blood, 136–137
    connective tissue, 137–138
    endocrine, 129–135
    human, autoantibodies in, 129
    renal, 135–136

Encephalitides, 104
Endocrine diseases, 129–135
Enterobacteriaceae, biochemical
    rapid identification, 41–49
Enterotube, improved, 44–45
Epstein-Barr virus, 105–125

Food, bacteria in, 158
Food and Drug Administration,
    regulation of in vitro diagnostic
    products, 7–10
Francisella, 88–90
Fungi
    immunological diagnosis of diseases
        from, 87–98
    results of chromatographic studies,
        167–179
    serology, 93–97

Gonorrhea, 93

Hepatitis, 103–104
Heterophil test, 105–125
Histoplasmosis, 97

Immunofluorescence tests
    for bacteria, 51–65

direct, applications in clinical and
    public health bacteriology,
    52–61
indirect, application in clinical and
    public health laboratory, 61
needs and future directions, in
    bacteriology laboratories,
    61–62
Immunology
    clinical laboratory, systems for,
        83–141
    diagnosis of bacterial and fungal
        diseases, 87–98
Impedance measurements, 31–32
Infections, viral, rapid diagnosis,
    99–104

Kidney, autoimmune diseases,
    135–136

Laboratory, state public health,
    training and regulatory func-
    tions, 15–22
Leptospira, 91
Limulus test, 34–36
Listeria, 52, 91

Microbiology
    increased role of regulatory agen-
        cies in, 1–22
    laboratory, trends in methodology,
        143–193
    radioimmunoassay, 147–152
    radiometry, 153–161
    role of computer, 181–193
Microcalorimetry, 32
Microorganisms
    chromatographic identification,
        163–180
    systems for detection and identifi-
        cation, 23–82
Minitek system, 46–47
Mononucleosis, infectious, labora-
    tory diagnosis, 105–125

Paracoccidioidomycosis, 96
Participants in conference, 199

Radioimmunoassay in microbiology,
    147—152
Radiometry in microbiology,
    153—161
Reagents, commercial, 95
Regulatory agencies, increased role
    of, in microbiology, 1—22
Regulatory functions of a state
    public health laboratory,
    15—22
Rickettsia, 90
Rubella, 101—102

Serology
    bacterial, 88—93
    fungal, 93—97
Sperm, antibodies to, 135
Sporotrichosis, 97
State public health laboratory,
    training and regulatory func-
    tions, 15—22
Streptococcus, 90—91
Summary of conference, 195—198

Susceptibility testing, 157—158
    antibiotic, 78—79
Syphilis, 91—93

Technology transfer, role of CDC,
    11—14
Toxoplasmosis, 102
Training of a state public health
    laboratory, 15—22

Virology, diagnostic, 99—104
    procedures, 100—104
Viruses
    Epstein-Barr, 105—125
    respiratory, 102—103

White cell metabolism, 159—160

Yeasts, chromatographic identifica-
    tion techniques, 164—165